'Professionals within the field of sexuality, whetl
sexologists, educators, academics, clinicians, etc., o
their careers that there is space for contract work. Despite possessing
the requisite education and theoretical background, many of these
individuals lack the business acumen required for success in this arena.
Even their colleagues, who may be facing similar challenges with their
own businesses, cannot always provide guidance. As a result, these
professionals are often left wondering how they can make a living as sole
practitioners in the sexuality field. It can feel like they are working in
isolation, with little support or understanding from those around them.

This is where the book at hand comes in. By bringing together a diverse
group of successful sexuality business owners, the author has created
a space for struggling or questioning business owners to receive much-
needed leadership and support. Through this collaboration, the book
provides hope and strategies for success, while also lending credibility
to the field of sexuality. It is a valuable resource for anyone seeking to
build a successful career in this complex and challenging industry. Thank
you, Dr. Wadley, for bringing these individuals together to support and
advance the sexuality business.'

Monique Howard, EdD, MPH, *Public/Sexual*
Health Consultant, Nonprofit Strategist

'Dr. Wadley and his colleagues create space for sexual and mental
practitioners to discuss the business components of our profession.
Undoubtedly, this is a wonderful contribution to the field.'

Kamilah Marie Woodson, PhD, *Professor of*
Counseling Psychology and Department Chair,
Human Development and Psychoeducational
Studies, Howard University

'We finally started the conversation about the integration of sexuality and
relational health studies and business. I am so proud of my colleagues for
initiating a formal conversation for us to learn and grow from.'

Carmelita Yvette Whitfield, PhD, *Associate Director*
of Community Health, Penn State University

The Professional's Guide to Sexuality Consultation

This book offers support and guidance to sexuality professionals who are looking at different strategies to progress their careers, accounting for the diverse jobs they can take on or create.

Bringing together contributions from the field of sexology, business, and marriage and family therapy, James C. Wadley combines elements of sexuality, business development, and entrepreneurship to help therapists consider their professional options. Chapters address topics such as how to navigate consultative opportunities in sex education, clinical work, counseling, coaching, supervision, research, non-profit and for-profit entities, volunteer experiences, and in academic settings. Professional contributions offer practical advice as well as personal reflections, with insights ranging from obtaining consultative positions, to starting one's own business, and using social media effectively.

Sexuality educators, counselors, therapists, healers, advocates, activists, researchers, policy makers, workers, and other consultants will find this book invaluable when navigating new ideas and professional paths they can take within the field.

James C. Wadley is a professor of the Master of Human Services department at Lincoln University. He is also Director of the Sex Therapy Program at Council for Relationships (Philadelphia, USA). He is the Editor-in-Chief of the *Journal of Black Sexuality and Relationships* and the founder and principal of the Association of Black Sexologists and Clinicians.

The Professional's Guide to Sexuality Consultation

An Exploration of Entrepreneurship, Strategic Planning, and Business Influence

Edited by James C. Wadley

Foreword by Marla R. Stewart

Routledge
Taylor & Francis Group

NEW YORK AND LONDON

Designed cover image: brightstars © Getty Images

First published 2024
by Routledge
605 Third Avenue, New York, NY 10158

and by Routledge
4 Park Square, Milton Park, Abingdon, Oxon, OX14 4RN

Routledge is an imprint of the Taylor & Francis Group, an informa business

Library of Congress Cataloging-in-Publication Data
Names: Wadley, James C., editor.
Title: The professional's guide to sexuality consultation: an exploration of entrepreneurship, strategic planning, and business influence / James C. Wadley.
Description: New York, NY: Routledge, 2024. | Includes bibliographical references and index. |
Identifiers: LCCN 2023026091 (print) | LCCN 2023026092 (ebook) | ISBN 9781032323657 (paperback) | ISBN 9781032323527 (hardback) | ISBN 9781003314660 (ebook)
Subjects: LCSH: Sex therapy–Vocational guidance–United States. | Sex therapists–United States.
Classification: LCC RC557 .P76 2024 (print) | LCC RC557 (ebook) | DDC 616.85/830023–dc23/eng/20230828
LC record available at https://lccn.loc.gov/2023026091
LC ebook record available at https://lccn.loc.gov/2023026092

ISBN: 9781032323527 (hbk)
ISBN: 9781032323657 (pbk)
ISBN: 9781003314660 (ebk)

DOI: 10.4324/9781003314660

Typeset in Sabon
by Deanta Global Publishing Services, Chennai, India

Contents

Acknowledgment

I would like to acknowledge my family for their patience and support during this long journey. I would also like to acknowledge my colleagues at Lincoln University, Council for Relationships (Philadelphia, USA), the Institute for Gender & Development Studies at University of the West Indies, and Keystone College for their contribution to this initiative. Finally, and most importantly, I would like to thank the contributors to this edited volume as you have started a long-needed business-related conversation for sexuality and mental health professionals.

Contributors

Editor

James Wadley, MBA, Ph.D., CST-S, is Professor in the Counseling and Human Services department at Lincoln University and Director of Sex Therapy for the Council for Relationships (Philadelphia, USA). As a scholar-practitioner, he is a licensed professional counselor and maintains a private practice in the States of Pennsylvania and New Jersey.

He is the founding editor of the scholarly, interdisciplinary journal, the *Journal of Black Sexuality and Relationships* (University of Nebraska Press). He is also the founder and Principal of the Association of Black Sexologists and Clinicians and his professional background in human sexuality education, educational leadership, and program development has enabled him to galvanize scholars and practitioners in the field of sexology across the world.

His research and publication interests include sexual decision making among young adults, masculinity development and conceptions of fatherhood by non-custodial fathers, and HIV/AIDS prevention. He has written undergraduate and graduate courses and authored 22 courses for the Master of Science in Counseling program for Lincoln University (PA). In addition, he recently co-authored 13 doctoral level courses for the Theological Seminary of Puerto Rico. In 2015, Dr. Wadley earned his NBCC-International Mental Health Facilitator certification after spending time with Rwandan therapists discussing the impact of genocide and trauma in the early 1990's. In 2016, he helped develop curricula and conducted a sexuality education course at the University of Muhimbili in Tanzania for the nursing and midwifery program. Later that year, he developed and taught an applied research methods course at Cape Peninsula University of Technology in Cape Town, South Africa. In 2017, Dr. Wadley's work and advocacy both domestically and abroad enabled him to complete his first documentary, *Raw to Reel: Race, Drugs, and Sex in Trenton, New Jersey*, which captures some of the challenges that emerge in addiction and recovery. Finally, in 2018, Dr. Wadley co-edited *The Art of Sex Therapy Supervision* (Routledge) which is a book devoted to the clinical experiences of supervisors and supervisees in the field of sex therapy. The book won AASECT's 2019 Book of the Year Award. In 2020, *The Handbook of Sexuality Leadership: Inspiring Community Engagement, Social Empowerment, and Transformational Influence* (Routledge) carves a new path for sexuality educators, counselors, and therapists in that it serves as an invitation for re-conceptualizing the consultative roles that sexuality professionals engage in. Finally, in 2021, Dr. Wadley and his colleagues (Reece Malone, Marla Stewart, and Mariotta Gary-Smith) edited the book *An Intersectional Approach to Sex Therapy: Centering the Lives of Indigenous, Racialized, and People of Color*. The book captures the professional experiences of BIPOC sexuality therapists and considerations offered to the clients they serve.

Dr. Wadley received his Doctorate of Philosophy degree in Education from the University of Pennsylvania with a concentration in Educational Leadership and Human Sexuality Education. He earned a Master of Science in Education degree in School Psychology from the University of Kentucky after completing his B.A. in Psychology from Hampton University. He holds a clinical postgraduate certificate from Thomas Jefferson University/Council for Relationships in Philadelphia. In 2020, Dr. Wadley also earned a Performance Leadership Certificate from Cornell University and an MBA from Keystone College in 2022 which has enabled him to help leaders engage in courageous and transformative dialogue about corporate social responsibility and strategic change. James is an AASECT Certified Sex Therapist Supervisor. These credentials and a wealth of domestic and international clinical experiences, have catapulted him to become one of the nation's best marriage, family, and sexuality clinicians and entrepreneurs.

Contributors

Shanae Adams, MA, LPCC, NCC, CIGT, is a Sexuality Professional from Denver, CO. She is a Taurus sun and moon and Virgo rising. While pursuing her Bachelors of Science degree at the University of Missouri, she served as a Sexual Health Advocate Peer Educator on campus. In this group, she discovered a passion for sexuality education and an adept ability to present these topics with a unique flair and an engaging personality. Shanae created HonestlyNae LLC to serve her mission of normalization, explanation, and melanated representation. Since its inception in 2017, HonestlyNae has conducted over 2,000 hours of education, presented at over 60 professional conferences, been featured on numerous blogs, podcasts, and educational outlets, and conducted several professional development seminars. HonestlyNae is a sought out voice for sexuality topics related to identity, pleasure, intersection, kink/fetish, sex work, trauma, and Queer, Trans*, Indigenous, Black, People of Color issues. Feedback for HonestlyNae includes, "Shanae presents these topics in a way that makes me feel seen and heard," and "It feels great to see

queer black femmes confident and knowledgeable about topics I struggle with." From this feedback, Shanae sought to create more intentional
community building to aid in her mission.

In 2019 The Chrysalis House LCA was co-founded to provide space
for transformation. The mission of The Chrysalis House is sex-positive
holistic radical affirmation and care. They accomplish this mission by
hosting joy-centered events, conducting education focused on financial,
emotional, and mental stability, and building a resource network of
clothes, food, and basic needs support. Their efforts were significant during the pandemic as they were able to provide 100 people with assistance.
They hope that as health rates improve, they can get back to in-person
events and activities but they have not let quarantine lessen their impact.
Their virtual community-building events have high attendance rates, and
they look forward to delivering these engagement opportunities offline.

Shanae received her Masters in Clinical Counseling from Adams State
University in 2020. She felt called to obtain this degree due to the com-
fortability and openness her participants experienced in workshops. It
was not uncommon for Shanae to be approached by attendees and asked
to hold space for their vulnerable feelings. She did her best but Shanae
felt there was a level of support the community asked of her that she
did not have to tools to deliver. Her private practice MAI Therapeutic
Services stands on three pillars: Manifest, Affirm, Intent. Shanae believes
her clients have the power to manifest a reality in which they can thrive
and that therapy can be an intentional space to focus on that work.
Shanae's role is to support and affirm her clients on that journey. Shanae
brings the same openness and engagement to her therapeutic clients that
she brings to her dynamic workshops. Her therapeutic modalities are
client-centered, somatic, and indigenized approaches. Many of her clients
struggle with millennial issues, identity difficulties, sexuality-related concerns, and feeling like they have more potential to reach. In the future,
Shanae hopes to educate future clinicians on sex-positive practices to create more opportunities for clients to be affirmed and supported on their
journeys.

Tanya M. Bass, Ph.D., M.Ed., MS, CHES, CSE, is a national award-win-
ning sexuality educator and a subject matter expert in the areas of health
equity and sexual health. She is an alumna of North Carolina Central
University's (NCCU) Department of Public Health Education and the
Center for Human Sexuality Studies at Widener University. She founded
the North Carolina Sexual Health Conference and is the lead instructor for Sexuality at North Carolina Central University. Much of her
work has been in collaboration with community-based organizations,
churches, academic institutions, and state and national organizations.
She co-chaired the 2014 National Sex Ed Conference and the 2020 and
2021 American Association of Sexuality Educators, Counselors and

Therapist (AASECT) virtual conferences. She is on the editorial board for the *American Journal of Sexuality Education* and wrote a chapter in *Handbook of Sexuality Leadership*.

Patti Britton, Ph.D./MPH, ACSE, is a well-respected pioneer in the field of sexology and is viewed as part of top leadership globally, having served on the Advisory Council for the World Association of Sexual Health, as past President of AASECT, and as a world leader of SAR. Britton is a nationally board-certified Clinical Sexologist and known as the "Mother of Sex Coaching." Britton is the Co-Founder of SexCoachU, the world's premier training and credentialing organization for sex coaches, and is the Co-Creator of its Business of Sex Coaching program. Her business acumen is derived from 30 years as a sexological entrepreneur, with mentorship/trainings by luminaries in coaching, entrepreneurship, and online business strategies and methodologies.

She is the author of the only SAR training manual, *Designing and Leading a Successful SAR* (Routledge Press, 2017), and the landmark *The Art of Sex Coaching* (2005). Britton has published hundreds of articles, book chapters, forewords, and five major books in sexology; she is a popular speaker to consumers and a seasoned professional trainer for her peers. Britton has hosted over 40 DVD programs on sexual enhancement. Her media record makes her a leading voice in sexology. Each year Dr. Britton conducts professional trainings or retreats, speaks at major events, participates in media interviews, guests on podcasts, is a featured expert at various virtual summits, and appears on camera for documentaries, webinars, and conference presentations. Her mentorship program can be found at: BrittonMastermind.com and her home website is: DrPattiBritton.com.

LaToya Cheathon, Ph.D., LMFT, is a Relationship Coach and Therapist, specializing in working with couples who desire to improve their relationships. She has completed her Master's Degree in Counseling Psychology at National University in Sacramento, CA, and Bachelor's Degree in Counseling Psychology and Theology from William Jessup University in Rocklin, CA.

LaToya has spent the last 14 years working in numerous environments, with many different populations, including working with children, teenagers, college students, and adults needing support in addressing trauma, substance abuse, criminal justice involvement, and homelessness, as well as a wide-variety of other concerns and challenges. However, she most enjoys working with couples having relationship concerns because she feels that the most effective way to help people work through difficulties in their relationship is to be able to sit with both partners, and learn about each person's perspective on the challenges they are facing.

LaToya is Level 3 trained in utilizing the Gottman Method, and utilizes this evidence-based model's techniques in her work with couples. In addition, LaToya is a Brainspotting Practitioner and she can provide this treatment during coaching sessions to help clients address individual life stressors.

During her coaching sessions, LaToya works to help couples develop the necessary skills needed to maintain sustaining love.

Candice Cooper-Lovett, Ph.D., LMFT-S, CST, is a wife, mom, and owner of A New Creation Psychotherapy Services LLC, a holistic group practice in the south Atlanta Metro Area. Additionally, she is the owner of Dr. Coop-Love a consultation, coaching, supervision, and mental health speaking business. Last, she is the owner of The Tantric MFT LLC which focuses on tantra/energy healing, and other spiritual services. A licensed marriage and family therapist and AASECT certified sex therapist, Dr. Cooper-Lovett is an AAMFT clinical fellow and approved supervisor. Additionally, she is a tantric/energy healer which expands the capacity of healing for individuals and couples. In addition, Dr. Cooper-Lovett currently serves on the advisory committee for AAMFT's minority fellowship program. She also serves as a reviewer for the *Journal of Interpersonal Violence*. Dr. Cooper-Lovett has almost 20 years of experience and specializes in trauma, specifically intimate partner violence, sexual abuse/assault. She also specializes in sexuality and sexual issues, as well as female sexuality and pleasure in both individuals and couples. Her work has contributed to peer-reviewed journals, as well as media articles and magazines. Dr. Cooper-Lovett has presented at many national conferences since her undergraduate career. Over the years she has also been on radio shows, podcasts, television, panels, workshops, CE trainings, and keynotes surrounding various topics around violence, marriage, sexuality and relationships, spirituality, infidelity recovery, clinical implications in working with African American youth, and mental health awareness in African American communities.

Melanie Davis, Ph.D., M.Ed., CSC, CSE, CSE-S, is a founding partner in the New Jersey Center for Sexual Wellness. She is a consultant and trainer in sexuality education, sexuality, and adjacent topics. She has taught graduate courses at Widener and Drexel Universities as well as Moravian Theological Seminary, and she has taught undergraduate courses at Moravian and Marymount Manhattan colleges. Dr. Davis is a certified sexuality counselor, educator, and educator supervisor through the American Association of Sexuality Educators, Counselors and Therapists (AASECT) and was named 2022 AASECT Sexuality Educator of the Year. She is the Our Whole Lives Sexuality Education Program Manager for the Unitarian Universalist Association and author of *Our Whole Lives Sexuality Education for Older Adults* and *Sexuality and Our Faith: A Companion to Our Whole Lives Sexuality Education for Grades 7–9 (2nd ed.)*. She has written chapters for *Handbook of Sexuality Leadership*; *The Art of Sex Therapy Supervision*; *How I Got*

Into Sex...Ed; and *Sex after...women share how intimacy changes as life changes*; as well as an abstract for the Association for Gerontology in Higher Education's *41st Annual Meeting and Educational Leadership Conference Abstract Book*.

Chasity Fowlkes, LMHC, MCAP, ICADC, CST, CDWF, is a Licensed Mental Health Counselor, Masters level Certified Addictions Professional, Internationally Certified Alcohol and Drug Counselor, Certified Sex Therapist, EMDR trained clinician, Certified Daring Way Facilitator, Gottman Level 1 Trained Qualified Supervisor for Mental Health Counselors. She is also a Certified Prepare-Enrich facilitator for dating, marital and pre-marital couples, and a trainer for others. Chasity is the CEO of this Practice and her new group practice Catalyst for Change Psychiatry & Counseling Services. Chasity has earned her Associate's & Bachelor's Degrees in Psychology and her Master's Degree in Counseling with an Emphasis in Professional Mental Health Counseling. Chasity is currently pursuing additional certifications in Substance Abuse and Sex Education. In addition to her educational accomplishments, Chasity is a three-time published author in the following books: *Best Selling Anthology Sex After Divorce: Been There, Done That & Had The Orgasm to Prove it!* of which she was the visionary author and with her chapter "Sex, Love & All The Bullshit in Between!" the 2019 Best Selling book *Brand New Me The Pursuit of Wholeness* with her chapter "A Quest to Feel Wanted" and the 2018 Black Therapist's Rock *A Glimpse Through the Eyes of Experts* with her chapter titled "Sex, Sexuality & Gender: The Unspoken Connection to Mental Health." She is currently working on several other book projects, helps helpers birth their books, and contributes her writing talents to several other magazines, platforms, and entities.

Chasity has over 19 years of experience in the helping field. She specializes in the following areas working with children, teenagers, adults, and couples.

Quantas Ginn, LMFT, CST, is a marriage and family therapist, who takes a systemic approach to therapy. He seeks to look at how the intersections of a client's life impacts who they are today. He helps them examine what role family, friends, and other life factors play in their life. Doing so, Quantas is able to help clients write the next chapter in their lives.

His aim is to create a safe® space for clients to process, learn, and make positive changes in their lives. Quantas works with individuals, couples, and families who wish to address emotional, relational, and identity conflict.

Stefani Goerlich, Ph.D., is an award winning author of *The Leather Couch: Clinical Practice with Kinky Clients* and it's advanced practice sequel, *Kink-Affirming Practice: Culturally Competent Therapy from*

The Leather Chair, Stefani describes herself as an expert on the edges and a bridge builder between the margins and the mainstream.

An expert in working with Gender, Relationship, and Sexuality Differences, as well as with those from minority religious traditions, Stefani is a Certified Sex Therapist, a Board Certified Diplomate of Sexology and an expert voice for *Cosmopolitan*, *The New Yorker*, *The New York Post*, *Shape*, *Women's Health*, *Marie Claire*, *The American Spectator*, and many more.

Stefani is a member of the teaching faculty at the University of Michigan Sexual Health Certificate Program.

Jennifer Litner, Ph.D., LMFT, CST, is a sexologist, a licensed marriage and family therapist, and a certified sex therapist. Dr. Litner is the founder of Embrace Sexual Wellness, a Chicago-based wellness center specializing in confidential, comprehensive care in sexual health through the integration of psychotherapy and educational programming for teens, parents, and healthcare professionals. Her expertise includes helping clients improve sexual functioning and satisfaction, loss of intimacy, and pain during sex. Her research explores comprehensive sexuality education and relationship satisfaction.

Sarah Martin, MA, CSC, is a Certified Sex Coach™, a graduate of Sex Coach U, and the Co-creator of the Business of Sex Coaching program. Martin honed her business skills during nearly a decade in corporate international operations roles before embarking on the entrepreneurial path. She has undertaken extensive training in business strategy and development focused on solopreneurs and entrepreneurs. Martin served as the Executive Director of the World Association of Sex Coaches from 2016–2021. She is a member of the World Association of Sex Coaches, the World Association of Sexual Health, and the Association of Somatic and Integrative Sexologists. Martin has a Masters in Sociology from the Graduate School for Social Research, Lancaster University, with a research focus on men and masculinities. She is one of a small number of academic experts on pickup artistry.

In her private practice, Martin provides her clients with a feminist, ethical alternative to pickup artistry called the Dignified Hedonist framework. She has worked with hundreds of clients worldwide through workshops, courses, and 1:1 coaching. Martin is the author of many articles, as well as the only book on Orgasmic Running, *Orgasmic Running: A Feminine Practice for Pleasurable Wellbeing* (2016). She was the co-host of the *Get Sex Smart* podcast and the host of the *Sexual Craftsmanship* podcast. Martin has been a featured guest expert on interviews for radio, podcasts, summits, and media, such as *BBC World News*, *Men's Health*, *The Guardian*, *The Irish Times*, *El Pais*, and *Sex Matters Magazine*. Her home website is: DignifiedHedonist.com.

Mary May, MFT, is a Leadership Strategist as an innovative thinker and an individual that creates personalized strategies to guide your success in your career. She helps women in corporate America go from being passed over to being promoted and well-paid.

Mary has practiced as an educator, relationship therapist, and program developer, with a solution focus on preventative intervention for over 25 years. She specializes in guiding individuals through emotional wounds that can lead to depression and anxiety that manifests from multi-layered trauma-responsive experiences.

In the last 12 years of her practice/professional career she has worked with individuals who are leaders in their space of excellence in their respective areas of expertise.

Marla Renee Stewart, M.A., (she/her) is a certified sexologist, sexual strategist, intimacy/relationship/sex coach, educator, speaker, and author. She is the owner of Velvet Lips, a sexuality education company that focuses on people to help them integrate seduction, develop their communication abilities, and enhancing their sex skills. As a faculty member at Clayton State University, she teaches Sociology and Women's and Gender Studies. As the Co-Founder of the Sex Down South Conference, Marla aims to bring diverse groups together to learn and share their experiences in the essence of being authentic and fostering sexual liberation across communities.

She currently runs two programs: the MEE program for people who want to have better relationships with themselves and with their lovers and the Sexcessful Business Coaching program to help business owners in erotic industries move their businesses past six figures.

Marla has studied human sexuality for over 22 years, has educated over 20,000 people in over 15 years, given over 1,000 workshops, and has served hundreds of clients in her private practice all around the world. She has had her influence in the media, as well; she has written over 200 articles, featured in over 100 magazines and books, and has been on over 80 podcasts and independent television shows. She was featured on Netflix's *Trigger Warning with Killer Mike*, VH1's *Love & HipHop Atlanta*, and has filmed as a sex expert for many more reality shows. In addition, she also sits on the Board for American Association of Somatic Sexology.

Her educational background is also robust. She received her BA in Psychology and minored in Human Sexuality/LGBT Studies from San Francisco State University. She gained her Master's Degree in Sociology with a concentration on Gender and Sexuality, while studying for Women's & Gender Studies certification at Georgia State University. She is currently in pursuit of her Ph.D. in Clinical Sexology from the Modern Sex Therapy Institutes.

She co-wrote her first book, *The Ultimate Guide to Seduction &* *Foreplay* (2020) with Dr. Jessica O'Reilly and wrote a chapter and co-edited *An Intersectional Approach to Sex Therapy*, released December 2021. She is now working on a book, *Black Feminine Dominance* (working title) that hopes to be released in 2024.

Sara Vogel, Ed.D., is a sexual empowerment educator who is on a mission to end sexual harassment and sexual violence on college campuses by increasing educational opportunities around sex, power, and pleasure. She is a trainer, presenter, speaker, and storyteller who weaves together research on sexuality, sexual violence, and gender to create relatable, funny, and engaging presentations around topics that often bring people incredible shame. As a survivor of sexual violence, these topics are incredibly personal to her. As an educator who has mentored college students for over 15 years, she finds joy and hope in hosting conversations that they are yearning to have.

Fredrick Zal loves the arts, outdoors, cooking food with friends, learning with differing perspectives, and practicing 茶道 (Chado, Japanese Tea Ritual). Thriving since cancer, Fredrick has found new erotic embodiment, dancing, hiking, and yoga when his body has capacity, teaching, and rigorously working toward a Ph.D. in Sexology.

Nurturing erotically marginalized people, Fredrick teaches consent, sexual attitudes reassessment, and sensuality with understanding of power differentials, socio-political impacts over the centuries, and ways to truly dismantle what may feel harmful acculturalizing systems. He implements meta-cognition, sexual world-view expansion, and value delineation through a multi-faceted lens of post-structuralism, post-colonialism, intersectionality, phenomenology, and embodiment.

Foreword

by Marla Renee Stewart, MA

I started my sexuality education business, Velvet Lips, in March of 2010. I only knew the basics back then of starting a business (registering a business, getting a bank account, put up a website, market myself) and in this particular industry, there wasn't anyone teaching about it that I knew of at the time. There were no other sex coaches that I knew of in the South, so I really had to venture out on my own to figure out how to make a name for myself. I read many business books, took courses, and did everything within my financial capability to try to build my business, but it wasn't enough.

I had clients from all walks of life. I had couples who had desire discrepancy, one person of a couple trying to learn new things to better their sexual relationship, and single folks who were coming into their own regarding their queerness or trying to figure out how to not be single anymore. The fact of the matter is, is that my clients were too far in between. Having clients now and then was a struggle. But then they told their friends who told their friends about me and my business started to pick up. Because my business picked up, I transformed my home into my office, seeing clients, and running workshops, all while going to graduate school, and working part-time at bars and restaurants to make ends meet. Because of everything that I was doing, my business was failing. No clients were walking in the door, I got fired from the last restaurant I worked at; I was dealing with racism at my graduate school preventing me from moving forward toward my dissertation; and I was flat broke, living off of my savings to make ends meet. I decided to rent out my two other bedrooms via AirBnB to make the rent, and I applied to a few universities to teach at.

From May 2015 to August 2015, I was in a tizzy trying to figure out what I was going to do with my life because I loved my work; I loved helping clients and I loved the message that I was bringing to the world. Tia, my business partner, and I had just started the *Sex Down South Conference* and I finally landed a job at a university right before the first conference took place. Taking on a full-time lecturing position meant that I had less time for my business and for the business that Tia and I created together. I wasn't earning much in my business, but for the first time in my life, I had a salary and it was more money than I had ever seen at $48k.

So, of course, when my boss asked me back for another full-time year, I said "yes" without hesitation, continuing to put my business on the back-burner and because I was contributing so much time at the university. Though Tia was at her job full-time, we were in a scramble to try to get something going on for the third year of our conference, which we cancelled and then made into a smaller one-day event. The pivot was a realization that our lack of time isn't going to make our dreams come true. So luckily, the following year, I moved to part-time at the university, moving to online classes only, and concentrated more on my businesses. I focused on the inner workings of business; from attaining sponsorships to marketing under SESTA/FOSTA to honing my negotiation skills, I gained a tremendous amount of knowledge. Then, my business started to flourish. I started to set myself up for success, got my dating and love life together by going to therapy, and then things took off.

I realized that I was starting to do something right in my businesses.

I got asked to be on television shows, podcasts, and I started to travel more. More organizations and universities invited me to do what I do best—teaching the masses and educating them about sexual liberation, communication, seduction, and enhancing their sex skills, all while being authentic—and the word was getting out that I was an incredible teacher, which enabled me to be asked back year after year. My popularity was ever-growing and I was making more and more money.

Because I set myself up for success, when the pandemic came, my business took off even more. I was interviewed by famed feminist Roxane Gay about my job and how she had come to realize how I'm an essential worker and I was privileged to tell her that the pandemic year had brought on my best year yet. My investment in a good butt pillow was key, along with feeling like a goddess in my pregnant body, and I came to be in a state of abundance that has grown each and every year.

But this didn't come out of nowhere. It took me over eight years to establish myself in this business as a leader, as a revolutionary, as an innovator in the sexual liberation movement before people finally started to see all of me.

My professional years keep getting better and better with an added element of a new child at the age of 41. Trying to have my dream of being a full-time mother and my business and be a good wife is not easy, but it is doable. There have been many meetings where my child is on the call with me or even times where I've had to rush to put him to sleep just so I can do a presentation, only to have him wake up in the middle of it. My wife and I's quest for in-home childcare the way we want has been difficult, and starting the process of having another child means that this life is going to take on a whole new set of challenges; but I'm ready for it.

Currently, I work 15–20 hours a week on/in my business and I'm proud to be over six figures and not being a therapist (I saw that my therapist charges my insurance more than $1k per session; sometimes, I think I might have gone into the wrong sect of this industry), but creating my own niche of being a Sexual Strategist. As a sexual strategist, I am able to combine the knowledge that I've learned over the last 22 years and has enabled me to set myself apart from others; weaving the knowledge of sex therapy, somatic therapy/bodywork, and comprehensive sex education to help me ensure that my clients are being sexually successful.

My investment in my business has also proved fruitful and other sexuality business owners and leaders have come to me for guidance to help them along in this journey for their businesses; in which, I'm proud that I have helped them also achieve six figure status. My *Sexcessful Business Program* tackles many of the tactics included in this book, and many of the stories from the program participants are quite similar to the journeys found here.

The fact of the matter is, there aren't a whole lot of resources for folks working in the sex and sexuality industry. We're constantly trading notes and figuring this thing out as we go, and as much as we try to listen to mainstream business ideology and practice, we have to realize that our businesses are going to need something different. We're constantly getting kicked off of social media platforms, banned from payment systems, demonized on *FOX News,* or sometimes getting attacked from organizations who fail to understand why we are doing this powerful and incredible work.

Wherever you are at in your business journey, just know that someone has probably gone through what you have gone through and finding the right supportive systems are necessary for you to get some help through those obstacles. This book is a great way to see the lessons that people have learned along the way, and I highly recommend that you take what you need to heart. The experiences of each person in these chapters are invaluable and whether the advice is about the journey, a specific tactic or technique, or envisioning yourself as a CEO who has big dreams and goals, you'll find value in this book.

Good luck on your journey and always remember that you don't have to do this alone.

xo, marla

Introduction

The COVID pandemic quarantine was difficult for many as it was an unanticipated global phenomenon that impacted families and communities. Confusion about wearing masks, vaccinations, distance between one another, and lots of information and misinformation made personal, relational, and familial decision making tough for everyone. As a sexuality therapist and practitioner, it was hard for me to think through how I could be "there" for my family as well as for my clients. Navigation through the unknown had a lot of physical, emotional, and even financial pitfalls. Up until the pandemic, I had never considered meeting with clients via telehealth but because of the high transmissibility of the virus, I decided to close my practice locations in Philadelphia and Pennington, New Jersey and begin to see clients from home.

Providing quality therapy from home while monitoring my youngest son's experience of first grade via Zoom was challenging. During the quarantine, it was difficult for my partner and I to get him to sit still, focus, and learn over the course of a school day and stay on task. Like many of his classmates, he wiggled in his seat and found himself easily distracted by our cat, Waffles, who would frequently approach him at his desk (dinner table) for a treat. I worked from my laptop and offered my clients scores of apologies for family disruptions and intrusions and they were all very grateful and compassionate as we continued to work through relational, emotional, and sexual health issues. I must confess that it was hard to get into a good rhythm of setting spatial boundaries while working from home.

When there was down time over the quarantine, I had a chance to reflect upon my clinical and business experiences in the field. As a family systems therapist, I had always subscribed to the notion of "everyone should be in the room" during therapy in order to change the system. *The system impacts individual and relational function and dysfunction. Good therapy is always done in person, face-to-face.* Because of the quarantine, that model could no longer work as, at one time, it was too dangerous to meet with clients in my office due to transmission of the virus. A few clinical questions that I pondered and processed were:

1. Will my clients be open to meeting with me via telehealth since there is no face-to-face contact?
2. How will telehealth impact the work that I do as a therapist? Will I be able to successfully help my clients reach their goals?
3. Will my Internet be able to consistently sustain telehealth platforms?

A few business-related questions that I pondered were:

1. Once I stop seeing clients in New Jersey or Pennsylvania at my office, should I continue to pay rent and will my landlord let me out of my lease?
2. Will I pay for storage for my furniture? Who will help me move furniture during a pandemic?
3. How will my revenue fluctuate once I see clients via telehealth and how will that change affect my income and quality of living?

I rented my Philadelphia office from 2007 until 2020. It wasn't all that fancy, but I had a lot of pride because it was one of the first spaces where I was completely independent as a professional. The cost of my space was $500 a month. My landlord never raised the rent and never made any repairs to the heating or air conditioning. My lease expired around 2009 and shifted to a "month-to-month" contractual arrangement. When I shared with my landlord that I wanted to close the office in 2020 due to the pandemic, he was grateful and thankful for the business relationship that we had over the years.

I packed up several boxes and gave away my office furniture to a local shelter. It was hard to let go of a lot of items (i.e., books, knick-knacks, pictures, etc.) because it felt like a chapter in my life had ended. I continue to mourn the loss of the space because like most things in life, change was unanticipated but necessary.

Similarly, for my office in New Jersey, my landlord was relatively lenient and understanding about shifting our lease agreement—but he still wanted his money. He reduced my rent from $950 to $475. I was still responsible for the balance of the lease (i.e., about $12,000) when I moved out in 2020, but I was given an opportunity to pay less for the foreseeable future. Without knowing the amount of revenue that I would generate, I accepted because I was able to save some money each month.

Between clients, helping my son with schoolwork, grieving the loss of my mother-in-law, and managing other aspects of the pandemic and quarantine, I thought about my lack of knowledge about business-related concepts while working from home. I wish that I had taken at least one business course just so I could understand a few concepts so that I wouldn't bump my head (figuratively) and have to pay a lot of money for my mistakes. With all the years of schooling and continuing education, I had no clue about developing a business. I felt disempowered but could only blame myself for not pushing myself over the years to learn more about the art of business.

Most clinical mental health, social work, wellness, and sexuality therapy programs do not have a business component as a part of their curriculum. It is unfortunate because there are many sexual and relational health/wellness practitioners who move into private or group practice; set up or work in a nonprofit; accept or create a "gig"; take an academic or administrative position at a college or university; become entrepreneurs; or engage in some sort of commercial practice. Sometimes when we (practitioners) are invited to talk about business or acquiring financial resources, we really struggle to find meaning and address the relationship that each of us have with money. For some of us, conversations about money are activating, triggering, or even traumatic due to our familial or relational history of financial abuse, abandonment, or neglect.

Given this deficit of our field, I wanted to create a written narrative space for sexual, relational, and mental health professionals to share their business-related experiences so that our field could begin to have more formal discussions about financial negotiations, management, marketing, and planning. This edited book is the contiunuation of a long-needed conversation about business that I hope is helpful to sexuality and mental health practitioners for the work that we do. The chapters are written from personal and professional experiences from various perspectives that invite us to think about the business-related decisions we make both as individuals and as a collective. I am grateful and proud of all contributors who shared their experiences and business-related decisions and I am looking forward to more voices sharing their work in the future.

1 Gig Work for the Sexuality Professional

James C. Wadley

Gig Work for the Sexuality Professional

For the past 100 years, adults typically viewed professional work from the perspective of having a particular kind of "standard" employment that is accompanied with some sort of formal contract (Connelly & Gallagher, 2004, p. 959). Typically, full-time employment is performed at a business establishment, requires between 30 and 40 hours of service, and sometimes offers a longer-term investment in training, pension/retirement, and possibly health insurance (Bidwell & Briscoe, 2009). Over the past 30 years or so, contracts between employers and employees have become more flexible and work spaces have become more agile in the way employers have sought and retained workers who performed certain tasks in a shorter amount of time (Cappelli, 1998). These "gig workers" typically don't require the company to make a longer-term investment via health benefits, pension, or training but merely serve in the capacity of meeting a specific need. Copranzano et al. (2023) suggest that "Gig work is labor contracted and compensated on a short-term basis to organizations or to individual clients through an external labor market." Because of contract flexibility, gig workers may work for a number of different companies at any one time and utilize a variety of skills to earn compensation and benefits. The amount of time devoted to one or more companies is negotiated and decided upon between the gig employee and the hiring company. Negotiations are completed in an effort to make it so that all parties are satisfied with the quality, duration, and outcomes of specified tasks. Gig work is becoming a popular professional route because of the opportunity for workers to get what they want out of a particular position.

Gig work continues to grow in the US and is becoming a major part of the labor fabric (Kässi & Lehdonvirta, 2018). It is estimated that there are around 27 million gig workers in the US and almost 90% of companies devote some tasks to gig professionals. Moreover, this trend extends globally and is also a part of labor markets in Japan and Europe (Yano Research Institute, 2016). What makes gig work enticing is the notion of shorter-term contracts and commitments. Uzaiko (2016) suggests that gig work is

DOI: 10.4324/9781003314660-1

a temporary professional position filled by an independent contractor for a brief term. Contracted work may offer the freedom and flexibility of roles, responsibilities, and expectations that professionals want that they may not get with full-time positions.

Cropanzano et al. (2023) suggest that gig work has several attributes that separate it from other professional positions. The first attribute is that because gig workers are not considered full-time employees, they may fall under the guise of being freelance contractors. Gig professionals typically don't subcontract out to other employees and more often than not, are not a part of a larger organization. As freelance professionals, gig workers may be considered to be entrepreneurs who maintain a business of contracting services or products for a particular company. The second attribute is that gig workers tend to fulfill expectations and complete contracts quickly and seemingly cultivate an array of jobs that require various skill sets. The third characteristic of gig work is that professionals do not receive a salary but are paid for completion of a particular task or project (Goods et al., 2019). The final feature of gig workers is that they sometimes sell their products or labor to agencies (Schor, 2020). Because of this arrangement of selling goods and services, Uzaiko (2016) suggests that gig work includes little to no attachment to employers or their establishments. The gig worker does not necessarily seek to establish deep connections or longer-term attachments to employers since contracts are specific and expectations may not require deeper relationships. Due to connections that are weaker and sometimes informal or unstructured contractual agreements, there is high likelihood of job turnover (Uzaiko, 2016). Thus, gig work can be expendable to a company and conversely, companies can be expendable to gig workers.

Doucette and Bradford suggest that gig work has evolved from a person having a primary job and a secondary (part-time) job to professionals taking on several gigs at any one time (2019). The increase in job opportunities that are time flexible, strong in pay, and for a short duration have contributed to a growing number of professionals migrating away from full-time work that may have time, spatial, and circumstantial boundaries compared to gig work. For example, a sexuality professional may take several days, weeks, or months to develop a curriculum but can still earn an income from teaching as an adjunct at a local college/university. In addition, since the person may only teach a course or two each semester, the professional may also have 8–10 clients as a part of a sexuality coaching business. None of the jobs overlap in terms of availability of service and each job requires a different competence and skill set. The jobs seemingly complement one another if the professional is able to manage time and tasks appropriately.

Given the interdisciplinary and entrepreneurial nature of the field of sexuality work, it is not uncommon for professionals to hold multiple short-term gigs. Because employers are able to meet goals and outcomes by hiring gig workers, the number of gig opportunities has continued to increase over the past 20 years in the sexuality field and there does not seem to be any evidence of any decline. Sexuality professionals may find an array of professional options that exist as therapists, counselors, educators, advocates, brand specialists, company ambassadors, administrators, consultants, and policymakers. The following section articulates some of the professional considerations that may influence gig work for sexuality professionals.

How might a company find someone to engage in gig work?

Finding someone who provides good work and is reliable can be a challenging task in the field of sexuality. Because of its value laden nature, sexuality work can be difficult for some professionals to manage. It is not uncommon for companies or agencies to hire someone and soon determine that there is an incongruence in expectations and skill sets. Similarly, the professional may also find themselves in a position where they are not offered the same kinds of supports as full-time employees and quickly become frustrated or fatigued. Referrals are usually a good option for companies to find gig workers.

Companies sometimes rely on referrals for specific work to be completed. Referral sources could speak to an employee's professional history as well as their emotional and relational skill set as it pertains to completing the work. It may be too costly and time consuming for companies to find someone in-house who has a particular skill set to complete a specific task. It may be easier to use company networks to hire someone from the outside than to locate or train someone from within.

Gig workers are now able to position themselves on websites or apps such as Upwork, Fiverr, Angie's, Thumbtack, Bark, Craigslist, LinkedIn, and other consultant platforms where they can advertise their services for free or low cost to companies. Companies may find it easier to navigate these sites and find gig workers with specific skill sets to complete a variety of tasks. For sites like Upwork, Fiverr, and Thumbtack, companies can post a particular job/gig and gig workers can bid on services to be rendered. Moreover, companies sometimes use social media platforms such as Facebook/Meta, Instagram, TikTok, or Snapchat to find sexuality professionals who are educators, marketers, brand ambassadors, or content creators.

How to become a gig worker in the field of sexuality

To become a gig worker in the field of sexuality, one must have an understanding of the professional landscape and be willing, knowledgeable, and skilled at a particular set of tasks. The professional would need to have an understanding about his/her/their professional priorities so that the gig work can be integrated into the work that one already does or plans to do. Too often, gig workers take on too many tasks for too many companies and are unable to fulfill expectations and assignments. As mentioned earlier, sometimes people will take on gig work as an addition to their full-time job. Other professionals may exclusively engage in taking on part-time jobs because of the flexibility and minimal attachment to a company. As entrepreneurs, gig workers could set up an individualized business plan so that they have clear objectives on how they want to use their talent and expertise. Here are a few components that could be included in an individualized business plan:

1. Executive summary. An executive summary highlights professional accomplishments and goals that enables the professional to seek a particular position.
2. Company description. The gig worker could be considered his/her/their own individual company. Thus, a company description may articulate the nature of the company as well as its intentions to serve potential employees. The description could offer a time scope (e.g., months/years of intended service, hours available, task specialty, etc.).
3. Products and services. This portion of the individualized business plan includes a description of the products, services, and possible outcomes that a gig worker provides.
4. Market analysis. A market analysis or environmental scan allows for the gig worker to assess the promotion of services, the audience who will benefit from services, as well as who might the existing competitors be who offer the same types of services.
5. Strategy and implementation. This portion of the business plan creates structure and intentionality around services or production by articulating how, when, and the rationale for each process to occur. Timeliness is crucial in that opportunities may be seized or rejected if professionals do not have a logical and systematic strategy for processes or events to emerge.
6. Financial plan and projections. In terms of compensation, some sexuality professionals have no idea about how to figure out what their financial goals might be or how long it might take to acquire those goals. A few questions to be considered might be:
   a. What is the compensation for this job?
   b. Is the compensation in alignment with other professionals who hold this position at the same or similar companies?
   c. How much money does the sexuality professional invest in maintaining a job? What supplies are needed? What training is needed? What other costs should be considered (i.e., transportation, parking, Internet, uniform, food expenses, etc.)?
   d. How long should the duration of the contract be in order to meet relative goals?

Once one establishes an individualized business plan, the professional should consider several other constructs before engaging in sexuality gigs. The following sections address Branding, Contract negotiations; Resignation, termination, and contract fulfillment; and Retirement considerations.

Branding

According to Evergreen and Sabarre (2019), branding has become increasingly important for consultants as they attempt to differentiate between themselves from the competition by sharing their "unique value proposition to the world." Similarly, Cakir (2008) offers that a brand may be a name, a term, sign, symbol, or design which aims to define product and services of a seller or selling group that is used to distinguish itself from others. Further, the brand may be words, layout, pictures or patterns that may also serve as indicators of a particular professional or purpose (Islamoglu, 2000). Branding involves who a professional is, the work or status generated from the professional, the product quality of what a professional does, and the professional's vision for what is to unfold. Inasmuch, branding is intricately woven with marketing and helps clients have a better understanding of both the professional and products offered. Evergreen and Sabarre (2019) suggest that one could consider branding by reflecting upon the following:

[Professionally], I am known for _____.
[Professionally], I want to be known for _____.

The authors further offer that the gap between the reality and one's goal is where/how branding efforts are focused. With the goal in mind (I want to be known for...), professionals should consistently build upon skills, competence, and resources. Evans (2017) indicates that branding involves being honest and engaging in ongoing self-assessment so that one fully understands his/her/their position among those who offer similar services, products, or status.

For the sexuality professional who engages in gig work, branding is crucial in that it informs potential employers and clients about who a professional is, the work that is engaged in, and possible (favorable) outcomes from investment or hire. Websites, social media, written/audio media, and other publications serve as branding agents that convey one's professional status and alerts constituents about one's skill set and availability. Yasar (2022) contends that branding is the formation of an identity for the [professional] or product and that allows constituents to identify with the provider or the service.

For sexuality professionals who subscribe to sex positive branding, they may attempt to differentiate themselves by offering that sex should be safe, consensual, and pleasurable. Use of images, symbols, word patterns, and suggestions that frame body positivity, individual agency, and healthy decision making may be integral to the establishment and maintenance of one's brand. Moreover, professionals may create opportunities for themselves by using a sex positive perspective or they may be able to engage potential employers who may offer jobs or gigs as a result of this viewpoint. Similarly, some sexuality professionals may create a brand that focuses on trauma, harm reduction, psychopathology, relational strain or fracture, or dysfunction. Like sex positive branding, these professionals may create opportunities for themselves in the form of workshops, retreats, or develop curricula that attempts to address fear, anxiety, or relational dysfunction. Sexuality professionals have to have a clear understanding about how they position themselves in the field and the audience they would like to engage with. For sexuality professionals seeking to find or create a gig with a particular company, understanding their own personal brand may impact contract negotiations.

Contract negotiations

What is unfortunate about the field of sexuality, relational health, and mental health is that it is a rare or an infrequent occurrence when providers are taught how to negotiate contracts. Supervision, mentoring, and formal education (i.e., graduate and postgraduate) typically involves clinical case processing, curriculum development, advocacy, teaching, or some other form of service delivery or product formation but does not include how sexuality gig workers negotiate contracts. When contracts are typically offered by prospective employers, some sexuality gig workers will take the first offer without articulating a counteroffer that offers more money, autonomy, benefits, or terms of severance. Once a gig worker receives a contract, it is not uncommon that the professional experiences "buyer's remorse" with the desire or opportunity to have asked for something more or different. Thus, there are a few items that sexuality gig workers should keep in mind when offered a job contract:

1. Goals—What might some of the reasons be for wanting a particular gig? Money? Status? Influence? Networking opportunities? Possible professional growth/advancement?
2. Contract duration—Short-term contracts may offer an opportunity to renegotiate at the completion of a task or time interval (i.e., 3, 6, 9, 12 months, 3 or 5 years, etc.). Longer-term contracts may foster stability and confidence in the job or gig.
3. Exclusivity (Non-compete)—An exclusivity contract or non-complete clause may indicate that the gig worker cannot work for a similar

company or provide a similar service while working for an employer. Sometimes exclusivity contracts extend beyond the time that the gig worker works for a particular company.

4. Benefits—Because of its transient nature and amount of flexibility, gig workers usually are not offered benefits (e.g., health related, vacation or sick pay, tuition remission, short- or long-term disability, retirement pay, etc.) but it is always helpful to inquire. If gig workers sign longer term contracts, they may opt to do so for less pay and merely work for benefits (see item #1).

Gig work can be challenging if the professional only works gig-related jobs. For example, if the gig worker is hired as a fee for service, outpatient therapist, and does not see mental or sexual health clients on a particular day, or if the client does not show-up for therapy, then the professional is not compensated. In contrast, if the person is a full-time employee, then the professional may continue to receive compensation even if the client does not show up. Compensation may also continue for the full-time employee in the event of sickness; usage of personal leave time; usage of vacation time; pregnancy; or loss of immediate family member. While gig work offers freedom and flexibility around work, they may prove to offer less stability when life happens (e.g., sickness, loss, or familial shift). If gig work is done during off hours when the professional is not at a full-time job, then they could continue to receive benefits from their full-time position and possibly earn extra money or compensation for engaging in part-time work.

It should be noted that while gig work offers time and task completion flexibility, gig work became a challenge during the COVID-19 pandemic because employers reduced the amount of contractual work opportunities. The pandemic was tough for many because gig work does not offer benefits or perks compared to full-time permanent work (Ahmad, 2021). Some employees had a difficult time securing gig work due to company layoffs and COVID-19 spatial and health restriction guidelines. Fortunately, when health policies were eased and quarantines were lifted, some companies opted to hire more gig workers rather than full-time employees to reduce the number of benefit packages.

Resignation, termination, and contract fulfillment

Due to gig work being a temporary employment opportunity, it is sometimes called "at will." The employer and the gig worker have the right to terminate a contract at any time for any reason. Whether the task is completed or not or the contract duration has lapsed or not, the employer and the gig worker can "walk away" at any time. Sometimes parties will create an avenue for service titration or transition work before parties depart from one another. Sometimes parties don't offer any notice of termination, severance, or shift in agreement(s). Gig workers and employers should be prepared for unanticipated or abrupt shifts to at will employment. Resigning is *always* an option for gig workers.

Retirement considerations

As mentioned earlier, engaging in full-time gig work offers many benefits for professionals who are interested in entrepreneurial activity. On the other hand, usually gig related contracts and relationships do not allow for corporate matching contributions towards retirement. In other words, when working full-time for a corporation, sometimes entities are able to match a certain percentage of earned money that is placed into a retirement account (i.e., pension, 401K, 403B plan). For example, when full-time employees allocate 3–7% of their salary to a retirement account, the respective company will add that same percentage to the account. Rather than saving 3%, the employee actually earns 6%. When the employee retires and reach a specified age (i.e., 65), they are entitled to all money that has been saved in the retirement account.

For gig workers, usually there are no matching funds issued. Gig workers are responsible for setting aside some money periodically and preparing for the season of their life when they no longer want or are able to work. If gig work includes short term contractually based assignments, gig workers may be at the mercy of their employer who can determine when a specific contract is finished. Thus, adequately planning for retirement is a necessity in that gig workers have to operationalize what "retirement" is and will look like as one ages. Retirement takes on many different forms including the complete cessation of work; reduced workloads over time; or the acquisition of part-time gig(s) to supplement retirement income/savings. It seems critical that gig workers have a clear financial plan and be mindful of how it may evolve over the years of professional work.

Conclusion

Sexuality gig work has become more prevalent over the years and there are an increasing number of employers who seek out professionals who want to complete specific tasks for shorter durations. Sexuality gig professionals need to be clear about their brand, scope of expertise, and goals so that they can secure opportunities that are in alignment with their professional positions. Sexuality training programs should consider adopting business courses into their curricula so that professionals can develop their own individualized business plan, engage in strategy development, and make decisions that allow them to maximize their skill sets. In addition, sexuality professionals who are interested in gig work should remain mindful of the "at will" nature of working at a company and be ready and prepared for abrupt shifts. This holds true for the gig worker who is a freelancer who can decide when and how services and products should be offered or withheld. While there may be several items for sexuality gig workers to consider, it seems like gig work is here to stay as it offers a myriad of positive opportunities for professionals as well as employers.

Questions for Reflection

1. What kind of gig opportunities have you had or are considering? How might the acquisition of those opportunities be influenced by your professional brand?
2. In your opinion, why might some sexuality professionals prefer gig work compared to full-time salaried employment?
3. What might your professional goals be if you exclusively did gig work? What are your thoughts about compensation and how much you might need in order to experience a sense of fulfillment? What might retirement look like for you and how will you prepare for it?
4. What has made it easy or difficult for you to negotiate professional contracts? Did you take the first offer and if so, how did you feel afterwards? Was the first offer fair and in alignment with other professionals who held that position?
5. If you are an employer, share the reasons why you would hire or not hire gig employees.

References

Ahmad, N. (2021). Gig workers: The new employment form in the new economy. *Ulum Islamiyyah, 33*(S4), 131–145.

Bidwell, M. J., & Briscoe, F. (2009). Who contracts? Determinants of the decision to work as an independent contractor among information technology workers. *Academy of Management Journal, 52*(6), 1148–1168.

Çakir, V. (2008, May). The relation of knowledge of made in between brand attitude and willingness to purchase. In 6th International Symposium Communication in the Millenium (pp. 769–783).

Cappelli, P. (1998). *New deal at work*. Boston: Harvard Business School Press.

Connelly, C. E., & Gallagher, D. G. (2004). Emerging trends in contingent work research. *Journal of Management, 30*(6), 959–983.

Cropanzano, R., Keplinger, K., Lambert, B., Caza, B., & Ashford, S. (2023). The organizational psychology of gig work: An integrative conceptual review. *Journal of Applied Psychology, 108*(3), 492–519.

Doucette, M., & Bradford, W. (2019). Dual job holding and the gig economy: Allocation of effort across primary and gig jobs. *Southern Economic Journal, 85*(4), 1217–1242.

Evans, J. R. (2017). A strategic approach to self-branding. *Journal of Global Scholars of Marketing Science*, 27(4), 270–311.

Evergreen, S., & Sabarre, N. (2019). Branding for the independent icnsultant: Basic to advanced. *New Directions for Evaluation*, 2019(164), 101–113.

Goods, C., Veen, A., & Barratt, T. (2019). Is your gig any good?" Analysing job quality in the Australian platform-based food-delivery sector. *Journal of Industrial Relations*, 61(4), 502–527. https://doi.org/10.1177/0022185618817069

Islamaglu, A. H. (2000). *Pazarlama Yonetimi (Stratejik ve Global Yaklasum)*. Beta Basum Yayum Dagitum, A.S.: Trabzon.

Kässi, O., & Lehdonvirta, V. (2018). Online labour index: Measuring the online gig economy for policy and research. *Technological Forecasting and Social Change*, 137, 241–248.

Schor, J. B., Attwood-Charles, W., Cansoy, M., Ladegaard, I., & Wengronowitz, R. (2020). Dependence and precarity in the platform economy. *Theory and Society*, 49, 833–861.

Uzailko, A. (2016). The gig economy's growing influence on the American workforce. *Business News Daily*, 30 June.

Yano Research Institute (2016). Survey on crowdsourcing platforms 2016. http://www.yano.co.jp/press/pdf/1569.pdf.

Yaşar, E. (2022). The effect of employer brand on workplace selection in the hospitality industry. *Journal of Tourism Theory and Research*, 8(2), 29–36.

2 Sexuality Education Consulting

The Things They Didn't Teach in School

Tanya M. Bass and Melanie J. Davis

Introduction

Graduate and certificate sexuality education programs typically afford opportunities to build knowledge in human sexuality, theory, curriculum design, teaching methods, and ethics, all of which are helpful to individuals who will teach and design curriculum. They do not, however, consistently prepare graduates to become successful sexuality education consultants. As a result, those who undertake consulting work must identify gaps in their knowledge and skills and find ways to address them in order to be both competent and competitive.

Using an informal mixed methods survey, the authors identified types of work being done by sexuality education consultants, their formal education, and the sources of their additional training. Also explored were consulting income, success stories, and responses to disappointments and disillusionment, which are common experiences in consulting practice. Analysis identified the importance of networking and community building. These and other findings should help sexuality educators discern whether consulting is a viable option for them. It may also help mentors, supervisors, and program developers create much-needed learning opportunities. As chapter co-author Melanie Davis recollects:

> After earning my doctorate in Human Sexuality Education and becoming an AASECT-certified sexuality educator, I partnered with a gynecologist and sex therapist to form the New Jersey Center for Sexual Wellness. My academic program didn't offer courses on business practices and I couldn't find many other independent sexuality educators, so I developed my own crash course in private practice. I set my session fee by trial and error, first under- then over-pricing my sessions, finally settling on an hourly rate, clients were willing to pay It's worth noting that the amount equated to half what people were willing to pay for sex therapy, but clients cannot submit sexuality education receipts for out-of-network reimbursement. There was no literature on how to run a private sexuality education consultation, so I interviewed sexuality

DOI: 10.4324/9781003314660-2

counselors and therapists and combined their suggestions with my expertise in setting goals and measurable learning objectives for each session. An occupational therapist taught me how to record session notes that would be useful for clients' at-home reference, and a medical office manager taught me how to secure records for HIPPA compliance. The process was daunting because no measure existed by which to measure whether I was doing any of this optimally.

This chapter is an attempt to ease the entry of other sexuality educators into consulting practice by providing information about their colleagues' experiences and advice.

Demographics

Race and Gender

Among the 23 people who answered an informal snowball survey, one identifies as Hispanic/Latinx, six as African American/Black, and 16 as white. One identifies as gender nonbinary, one as "other," 17 as women, and four as men. Their ages range from to 24 to 70, with a median age of 43.

Educational Background

The authors did not list higher education as a qualification for participating in the survey, but seven respondents hold doctorates, 12 hold master's degrees, and one holds a bachelor's degree. Several respondents hold degrees in multiple specialties, with undergraduate and graduate studies representing 10 degrees in psychology; 12 degrees in human sexuality, sexuality education, queer or women's studies; four in public health; four in social work; and one each in education, poetics, bioethics, Indigenous women's studies, business, criminal justice, semiotics, anthropology, Spanish, history, liberal studies, health education, theology, youth development, communications, and biological sciences.

Sexuality Education Consulting Experience

The respondents have been sexuality education consultants between two to 30 years, with a median of seven years. They have served in the following roles:

- Brand management/ambassador.
- Business management advisor.
- Christian-specific consultant.
- Coach for individuals and families.
- Conference presenter.

- Consumer program presenter.
- Curriculum developer.
- Disability counselor and resource curator.
- Educator for a clinical practice.
- Educator for a health department.
- HIV research for PhD and publications.
- LGBTQIA+ content creator.
- Non-profit consultant.
- Policy advisor.
- Private practice sexuality educator.
- Professional development provider for educators, social workers, healthcare professionals, medical students.
- School and school district consultant.
- Sexual wholeness mentor.
- Strategic analyst and planning advisor.
- Supervisor.
- Teacher/guest lecturer.
- Thought leader.
- Training designer.
- Website content creator.

Income from Sexuality Education Consulting

Only three respondents reported being able to support themselves (or their families) on their sexuality education consulting income alone. Consulting is the primary but not sole source of income for six respondents, and it provides supplemental income for ten respondents. Eight respondents described consulting as a side hustle, which is part-time work completed outside hours spent on one's primary job (e.g., a public-school health teacher might have a side hustle delivering sexuality-themed workshops in their community). The survey did not ask how many hours respondents spent in any of these capacities.

Four respondents reported a "good year" to be one in which they earn $500–$1,000 from consulting; four said $1,000–$5,000; three said $5,000–$10,000; six said $10,000–$50,000; and four said $100,00 or more. Among those earning $100,000 or more, three reported it as their primary source of income, and one considered it supplemental income.

Post-Academic Training

As this chapter's title indicates, the authors sought to learn what types of knowledge and skills sexuality education consultants needed to gain after completing formal academic programs. Two areas were explored: training in sexuality and training in business management. Sexuality training was included because educators come to the work from diverse backgrounds without a common curriculum. The survey addressed business acumen because consulting success requires planning, marketing, assessment, training, pricing, management, budgeting, and accounting, yet sexuality education programs typically lack comprehensive coverage of these skill sets. This failure to address the proverbial elephant in the room regarding business management disempowers sexology professionals, especially educators who cannot refer to requirements spelled out for licensed professionals.

The authors started with the premise that before post-academic training is undertaken, a professional must recognize that they have more to learn.

Sexuality Educator Dispositional Humility

Typical academic and certificate programs in human sexuality offer a foundation for sexuality educators' scope of practice as defined by the American Association of Sexuality Educators, Counselors and Therapists (AASECT), which states that the work includes, but is not limited to, the following:

> teach and train about a range of topics, including but not limited to sexual health; sexual and reproductive anatomy and physiology; family planning, contraception, and pregnancy/childbirth; sexually transmitted infections; gender identity and roles; gay, lesbian, bisexual, and transgender issues; sexual function and dysfunction; sexual pleasure; sexual variation; sexuality and disability; sexuality and chronic illness; sexual development across the lifespan; sexual abuse, assault, and coercion; and sexuality across cultures. Sexuality educators may teach in the classroom at the elementary, secondary, and higher education levels. They may also provide education for groups of children, adolescents, or adults, training for professionals, and outreach and education in community-based, healthcare, corporate, and faith-based settings. Sexuality educators also may design and conduct workshops, courses, and seminars; contribute to the sexuality education literature; develop curriculum; plan and administer programs; deliver lectures; and provide one-on-one client education sessions.
>
> (AASECT, 2022, 11, AASECT-Certification)

Consultants need additional education to prepare them for tasks including how to set up and run a business, negotiate contracts, run meetings, consult with clients, create products and services, protect their intellectual property, engage and manage subcontractors, design and lead trainings, write and deliver speeches, write grant proposals, work with human services providers and agencies, craft policies, and do advocacy work. These skills are not addressed by AASECT's required core knowledge areas for certification.

One key to acquiring that necessary knowledge is *sexuality educator dispositional humility*, which is the willingness to acknowledge that one has more to learn. The term is defined as follows:

> ...sexuality educator dispositional humility requires the awareness of self and the willingness to learn as factors that ensure a more accurate self-assessment and willingness to seek professional development.
>
> (Bass, 2021).

When asked if "dispositional humility" was a characteristic they embodied, respondents' answers included:

- "We all need to stop and re-evaluate how we do things periodically. Even if we hold particular expertise, there is always an opportunity to learn from a new set of eyes. I have tried to keep myself open to new approaches and resist the temptation to continue utilizing the same techniques because they are familiar and/or have 'worked' in the past."
- "Kinda wondering if it's true humility to say you're humble, lol, but I'm actually always trying to learn something new—not just apply old information in new ways but to see what new information exists, because I think it's a misperception to believe we know all there is to know..."
- "Yes! I do this all the time because it keeps me innovative and evolving in the field."

Unlike those who teach calculus or Latin, sexuality educators must monitor evolving scientific knowledge and cultural norms. The discipline itself is evolving, with many educators working to dismantle white supremacy culture within the profession and the institutions in which sexuality education is provided. In addition, educators are developing new forms and standards of practice, such as a model for sexuality educators' ethical decision making (Nevers, Eastman-Mueller, & Oswalt, 2022). The survey response encouraging professionals to re-evaluate their body of sexuality knowledge also applies to running a consulting practice. Pricing should be reassessed to reflect expertise gained over the years. Educators also benefit by staying current on presentation and communication technologies as well as social media marketing approaches such as Instagram, TikTok, and the role of market influencers.

Training in Sexuality

Every respondent reported gaining some type of sexuality training or other form of education outside of or after completion of their academic training.

Conferences were identified as key learning opportunities, with respondents mentioning the following hosting organizations most often:

- AASECT.
- Center for Sex Education.
- Maine Family Planning.
- Society for the Scientific Study of Sexuality.

Other training opportunities respondents identified included:

- AASECT-approved programs and trainings.
- AASECT-approved individual and group supervision.
- Books and journals.
- Graduate courses.
- Independent study.
- Institutes providing degrees and certificates in sexuality education, counseling, coaching, and therapy.
- Master Certified Health Education Specialist (MCHES) self-study and conferences.
- Our Whole Lives Sexuality Education Facilitator Training through the Unitarian Universalist Association and United Church of Christ.
- Peer-to-peer mentoring.
- Reproductive healthcare organizations.
- Sex Ed Lecture Series.
- Sex Education Alliance chats.
- Sexual Attitude Reassessments (SARs).

Business Training

Seven respondents have not had business training, and some others respondents conflated training in their professional specialty with training in business. Excluding the latter group's answers to this question from analysis, the types of business training respondents reported taking include the following:

- Basic business skills for sexuality professionals.
- Business conferences.
- Coaching from a colleague.
- Coaching from a business specialist.
- Facebook groups on business consulting.
- Sex Education Alliance activities.
- Six Boxes Performance Training.
- Workshops on elements of running a business.
- Undergraduate and graduate studies in Business Administration and Business Management.

When asked what type of business training respondents would recommend to others seeking to become consultants, respondents' answers included:

- "I learned my business skills on my feet, through trial and error. I learned grant-writing skills by studying successful grant applications."
- "I've had no business courses or trainings specific to consultation work yet, though it would be helpful! I've mainly informally collaborated with consultants or small business owners to better understand the process of business ownership, marketing, etc."
- "Two books that have helped me, as someone with multiple minority identities, are *Linchpin*, by Seth Godin, and *We Should All Be Millionaires*, by Rachel Rogers."
- "If you have a business mind, you can apply general business training to this work. I do a lot of consults with colleagues."
- "Networking with other consultants to gain insights. This is a specialized sub-field, which I doubt traditional business coaching/training knows how to address."
- "Business and leadership courses."
- "Training in business structuring (tax identification, etc.) and liability."
- "How to use bookkeeping software and what you need to know about taxes."

Entrepreneurship

Eighty-three percent of survey respondents answered Yes to the question, "Do you consider yourself an entrepreneur?" which the authors defined as an innovative individual who organizes, manages, and operates an independently owned business or businesses. Entrepreneurs typically have high self-efficacy and a desire to achieve (Gielnik, Krämer, Kappel, & Frese, 2014), and entrepreneurship is a way of thinking, i.e., a multidisciplinary process of creating economic and social value in the face of uncertainty and limited resources (Klein & Bullock, 2006). Financial insecurity is one risk associated with entrepreneurship, given that income may ebb and flow unless professionals generate consistent cash flow and have predictable expenses. That said, entrepreneurs do not necessarily need large amounts of capital if they remain alert to profit opportunities (Klein & Bullock, 2006; Gielnik, Krämer, & Kappel, 2014). These opportunities may be identified by monitoring requests for proposals, calls for speakers, advertisements for curriculum and policy developers, requests for workshop or seminar presenters, job posts for adjunct teaching, and calls for journalists, bloggers, podcasters, and product reviewers. Sexuality education consultants who innovate and seek out these opportunities can stand apart from other consultants, which can mean the difference between a successful consultancy and mere maintenance of a small practice.

Experience in the profession is another aspect worth considering. One might assume that the more years someone does consulting, the greater their odds of identifying new business opportunities; however, they may experience "functional fixedness"—or being in a rut—that makes it hard to recognize new ways of operating (Shepherd & DeTienne, 2005, as cited in Gielnik, Krämer, Kappel, & Frese, 2014). The possibility exists that less-experienced consultants may be better able to piece together pieces of information than more-experienced consultants because their ways of thinking are not fixed (Gielnik, Krämer, Kappel, & Frese, 2014). This bodes well for sexuality education consultants with less than the median seven years' experience among survey respondents.

Creativity is a common characteristic of entrepreneurs, since it allows individuals to combine pieces of information and generate ideas for new products or services, which may then lead to more business opportunities (Gielnik, Frese, Graf, & Kampschulte, 2014; Shane & Venkataraman, 2002; as cited in Gielnik, Krämer, Kappel, & Frese, 2012). Sexuality education consultants surveyed for this chapter expressed a great deal of creativity and opportunity-creation, citing successful ventures including founding annual conferences; creating online sexuality education programs generating passive income; collaborating with jails and detention centers; writing innovative curriculums; teaching clergy how to use the power of the pulpit in sexual health promotion; and providing a Pride Month program while dressed in drag. The survey did not inquire about fees negotiated for these projects, so it remains unknown whether a correlation exists between creativity and income.

An interesting comparison can be made between the 83% of respondents who consider themselves entrepreneurs and the 4% who have at least some business training. The small sample group indicates entrepreneurial sexuality education consultants may be capitalizing both on their personality styles and their ability to create and take advantage of opportunities to learn business skills and to foster an entrepreneurial attitude. Answers remain elusive as to whether entrepreneurship is a teachable skill rather than an essentialist personality characteristic (Klein & Bullock, 2006; Lope and Abdullah, 2009), although a study of 17,277 pairs of twins (about half monozygotic [identical] and half same-sex dizygotic) in the United Kingdom found relatively high heritabilities for entrepreneurship, with little impact correlated to family environment and upbringing. The findings suggest genetic factors relate to why people engage in entrepreneurial activity (Nicolaou, Shane, Cherkas, Hunkin, & Spector, 2008).

A small study on twins conducted in the United States (Shane & Nicolaou, 2013) found that genetics affect the income earned by self-employed individuals. The study also found a genetic influence on agreeableness, openness to experience, extraversion, and self-employment income. While not all self-employed people consider themselves entrepreneurs, the findings reported in this chapter indicate the utility of the same traits.

The authors posit that while business skills are teachable, entrepreneurial drive is likely to be inherent. As Dutta (2017) noted:

> Just like tone-deaf individuals cannot sing, a person without charisma, integrity, honesty, vision and courage cannot become an entrepreneur... Entrepreneurship is an art, not a science. It is a set of innate traits that is perfected with time through learning and experience. Not everyone can be a good entrepreneur just like not everyone can be a good actor. Nothing can turn a follower into a leader.

It bears noting that while 83% of survey respondents identify as entrepreneurs, that identity is not a requirement for success; rather, interpersonal skills are the essential quality that facilitate professional connections that help professionals overcome many challenges.

Collegiality

One respondent noted the challenge of staying up to date on subject matter if one lacks access to institutional resources. These resources can range from academic and medical libraries, research assistants, statistical analysts, discounted or free course and training registration, regular access to colleagues, event planners and publicists. This is an important issue given the generally low pay sexuality educators many survey respondents reported as under $10,000 annually. The financial burden of training and journal subscriptions can increase the risk of professionals becoming obsolete and/or doing harm by perpetuating outdated information. Supervision, mentorship, and role modeling can provide ways to get around some of that lack of economic and academic privilege only if leaders have the business acumen to provide business-specific advice (Davis & Glick, 2020). This goes hand in hand with the need to build social capital through social relationships nurtured over time, which allows individuals to achieve interests and goals they could not achieve on their own (Davis & Glick, 2020).

Answers to multiple survey questions indicated respondents' need for and commitment to networking and collaboration as ways to build knowledge and to access opportunities they lacked access to on their own. As one person noted, "Networking and relationship-building are EVERYTHING. Surround yourself with talented people who get results!" The authors infer that this respondent may have connected results with the attainment of goals and/or income.

Due to the common practice of using professional forums to promote one's successes rather than failures, emerging professionals may lack role models for dealing with the inevitable struggles of consulting practice. For this reason, the authors asked questions about disappointment and disillusionment.

Disappointment and Disillusionment

Sexuality education consultants must learn to manage both disappointment and disillusionment. As defined by the authors within the survey, disappointment is the emotion felt when a strongly held expectation is not met, while disillusionment is a feeling of disappointment arising from the realization that something is not what it was expected or believed to be. These emotions are not typically addressed in academic programs but are part of consulting: deadlines are missed, proposals are declined, contracts are unfair, working relationships become unmanageable, goals are unmet, and income may be far lower than anticipated. Emerging sexuality educators are often risk averse because they fear failure; however, that fear may lessen if feelings of disappointment and disillusionment are explored with peers and colleagues. This type of discussion can help educators reconceptualize disappointment not as failure but rather as a "loss of the fantasy of stability" (Clancy, 2012). Viewed this way, possibilities remain open, imaginary ideals can be replaced by realistic goals, and consulting may remain a professional option.

The authors queried sexuality education consultants about these aspects of their profession to gain insights into how emerging sexuality educators might better prepare for the realities of consulting work. Many of the respondents indicated that much of the disappointment they experienced was due to compensation and the low value placed on their expertise for consultant services. When asked to give an example of a disappointment they experienced as a sexuality education consultant, respondents' answers included:

- "I am consistently disappointed at how often organizations don't think they need my expertise."
- "I think I was most disappointed when an organization with whom I have been working closely to prepare and deliver an amazing event cancels it due to lack of interest or simply low registration. It's hard in those moments to not internalize such things."
- "I think some of the biggest disappointments that I've had to date were that other sexuality entities do not value the work that we do in this field and are often the first ones to compensate us unfairly for the work and labor that is being requested."

Consultants must prepare themselves for disappointment while remaining eager to create new opportunities, make adjustments, and use each opportunity to make plans for future successes (Klein & Bullock, 2006). At the same time, they would be well served by looking forward to success, which can come in myriad forms.

Success Stories

Survey respondents reported the following success stories, which indicate that success is not necessarily measured in monetary terms:

- "My most successful experience was working with a tribal community to learn about different cultural aspects of sexuality education and training. This was successful in my opinion because it expanded my understanding of this community's needs, their supports and barriers, and how I can better serve this community and others in the future. I find any increase in understanding of cultural diversity and perspective-taking skills to be beneficial lessons."

- "I think the current project I'm working on is probably my most successful to date, based on the criteria of a) doing work I enjoy; b) being paid the amount I asked to be paid without haggling; and c) being able to bring my unique skills and perspective to it. I think the biggest lesson I've taken away is that I am more successful when I am clear about what I bring and don't compromise that to try and fit within the client's limited scope, even if they believe we have the same or similar work objectives."

- "My most successful sexuality consulting experience was in the development of a three-part racial justice for sexuality professionals training course. What I learned in the running of it the first time allowed me to adjust and change the program for subsequent times that it was run."

- "I learned more about how people adjust to new knowledge and how to give more space for them to adjust in that knowledge. I also learned that people do not know the racist history of the sex education specialty. I consider the weekly lectures I organize, the Sex Ed Lecture Series, to be my best consulting success. It is richly rewarding to me, even for weeks when I lose money, because I get to network and learn from so many interesting experts on a vast array of topics. It is successful because it does fairly well financially, and I have created an ethical model—one in which speakers are compensated not only for their time delivering lectures but also for orders of their recordings."

- "I developed a curriculum for a nonprofit client, and it was really gratifying to see the work come together into a finished product. I enjoyed the back-and-forth feedback process with my client, knowing that we were collaboratively improving the curriculum. One thing I struggle with as a consultant is not always getting positive reinforcement like I used to from a supervisor, so it made me feel successful to receive praise for my work and know I was meeting or exceeding their expectations."

Notable among these responses is the pride and emotional rewards consultants receive by meeting or exceeding their own or their clients' expectations. The balancing act between disappointment and reward may be eased through shared wisdom, as professional colleagues learn from each other.

Shared Wisdom

When asked what wisdom they could offer someone who is considering starting a sexuality education consultancy, respondents offered the following:

- "Set your fees higher than you are inclined to, and express willingness to negotiate. Most clients negotiate, which results in you getting closer to what you want."
- "Do good work and be guided by your vision, not the client's and definitely not the money."
- "This isn't an easy way to earn an income."
- "Figure out what you are passionate about, take note of your skills, hone your skills, research your target market, and access your market in a way that works for them geographically, culturally, and fiscally."
- "Your client may or may not see you as the ultimate expert; either way, demonstrate that you are also a learner and that you value insights your client can provide to you."
- "Keep to your lane...do the work you were doing without constantly comparing it to what other people are doing...which can often serve as a distraction from what we are doing ourselves."
- "Own your ignorance. You are never going to know it all, and pretending will only cause pain."
- "Be patient and don't expect to be in demand right away."
- "When working with young people, realize they are not giving you a hard time; rather, they are having a hard time. Understand people have invisible barriers and be compassionate—you don't know what someone else is experiencing."
- "Persevere and don't give up when facing obstacles."
- "Don't be afraid to charge high rates: you'll be surprised at how easily folks agree, and you deserve to earn a decent income!"
- "Have fun. This is a small profession where most everybody knows most everybody. We are not in competition with each other."

Conclusion

As the results of an informal survey illustrate, sexuality education consultants are doing a range of work that requires creativity, innovation, networking, collaboration, and risk-taking. By and large, sexuality consultants are not making significant amounts of money, yet their success stories indicate the commitment, enthusiasm with which they approach their work, as well as the satisfaction it brings them.

The consultants agree on the need for continuing sexuality education beyond one's academic course of study, as well as the need to learn business management skills. The findings also emphasize the importance of networking and community building. These findings should help sexuality educators discern whether consulting is a viable option for them. It may also help mentors, supervisors, and program developers create much-needed learning opportunities.

Questions for Reflection

Education And Training

What are your career goals? What suits your budget, timing, capacity, philosophy?

Are You An Entrepreneur?

Do you want to work independently or work for an organization full time? Do you enjoy developing new products and services? Emotionally and financially, can you afford to take risks?

Professional Disposition

Do you believe you have more to learn? Can you practice dispositional humility and take existing knowledge deeper by exploring new ways to apply it?

References

American Association of Sexuality Educators, Counselors and Therapists (2022). Certification overview. AASECT.org https://www.aasect.org/aasect-certification

Bass, T. M. (2021). *Examining the professional disposition among community-based sexuality educators.* (Doctoral dissertation, Widener University).

Clancy, A. (2012). *The organization of disappointment.* (Doctoral thesis, University of Bath).

Davis, M., & Glick, K. (2020). Networking, mentoring, collaborating, and risk-taking: A four-strand approach to sexuality leadership. In James Wadley (Ed.), *Sexuality leadership, empowerment, and consultation.* Melbourne, Australia: Routledge/Taylor & Francis.

Dutta, A. (2017). Can you learn entrepreneurship or are people born with it? Entrepreneur India. https://www.entrepreneur.com/en-in/leadership/can-you-learn-entrepreneurship-or-are-people-born-with-it/292622

Gielnik, M., Krämer, A.-C., Kappel, B., & Frese, M. (2014). Antecedents of business opportunity identification and innovation: Investigating the interplay of information processing and information acquisition. *Applied Psychology, 63*(2), 344–381.

Klein, P., & Bullock, J. (2006). Can entrepreneurship be taught? *Journal of Agricultural and Applied Economics, 38*(2), 429–439.

Lope, Z. A. and Abdullah, A. S. (2009). Exploring the entrepreneurial mindset of students: Implication for improvement of entrepreneurial learning at university. *The Journal of International Social Research*, 2(8), 340–345.

Nevers, J. M., Eastman-Mueller, H. P., & Oswalt, S. B. (2022). Ethical decision-making for sexuality educators: A new model. *Sex Education*. doi: 10.1080/14681811.2021.2020089

Nicolaou, N., Shane, S., Cherkas, L., Hunkin, J, & Spector, T. D. (2008). Is the tendency to engage in entrepreneurship genetic? *Management Science*, 54(1), 167–179. https://doi.org/10.1287/mnsc.1070.0761

Shane, S., & Nicolaou, N. (2013). The genetics of entrepreneurial performance. *International Small Business Journal*, 31(5), 475–495. https://doi.org/10.1177/0266242613485767

3 Developing and Implementing an Intentional Framework for Quality Hires and Sustainable Growth in Sexuality Business

Jennifer Litner

Introduction

A brief Internet search using keywords "how to hire as a sexologist" leaves little to be desired. Nearly all results are focused on continuing education in sexology or resources for prospective clients. So, *where do professionals learn how to effectively grow their business and hire quality candidates?*

To my knowledge, this is the first publication of its kind to focus on the hiring needs for sexuality professionals. In this chapter, sexuality professionals include sexuality consultants, sex educators, sex researchers, sex therapists, sex counselors, sex workers, and other health professionals working in the field of sexuality (Certification Types, 2022; Pillai-Friedman et al., 2014). While many publications about hiring and entrepreneurial growth exist, they do not center the specific and unique needs that sexuality professionals have. For example, sexuality professionals need business practices that consider their personal safety and wellbeing given our history of being criticized by the media and people who are resistant to sex-positivity (Freire, 2018; Lazkani, 2021; Sri Kantha, 2021; Tiefer, 1994). We know that sexuality professionals are likely to experience unwanted sexualization solely based on our profession (Levand & Canan, 2018). In the book *Bonk*, Mary Roach (2008) described researchers having people label them as perverts and concluding that they are fulfilling their own erotic interests when researching sexual functioning (pp. 12–13). Along with ridicule from professional colleagues, sex researchers may also experience what Roach (2008) refers to as the "cringe factor" from friends and family (p. 17). Because of this unwanted sexualization and criticism, professionals ought to be thoughtful about the people they hire and the systems they have in place to safeguard their businesses.

Unfortunately, few business coaches who have a keen understanding that sexology exists. Thus, sexuality professionals who wish to work closely with a coach may end up spending more time educating their coach about their field. This can be a costly burden both mentally and financially. As a result, sexuality professionals are limited in entrepreneurial support and resources for growing our business. Some professionals rely on their peers or search

DOI: 10.4324/9781003314660-3

within their social network of individuals who have experience working for corporations, in human resources, or business coaching to help them along the way. Others, figure it out as they go.

The reality is that sexuality professionals are not given a roadmap when it comes to building their business and hiring qualified candidates. As a result, sexuality entrepreneurs may be prone to feeling lost and unsure of where to begin when it comes to hiring, which could lead them to delay business expansion or approach hiring in nonstrategic ways that burden their businesses. Throughout this chapter, I use the term 'sex-preneurs' to refer to any sexologist or entrepreneur in the field of human sexuality. This chapter is for any sex-preneurs who have ever felt lost when expanding their business and wish they had a framework for developing a sustainable hiring practice. My perspective is influenced by my personal identities as a white, queer, partnered, Jewish, able-bodied, cisgender woman and business owner in an urban, progressive climate. In this chapter, I cover how to get in the right mindset for expansion, identifying business needs, developing a thorough, value-congruent process, determining which avenues to use for promotion, and curating a team with intention. First and foremost, we must get clear on how our attitude can inform the direction of our business.

Getting Real with Ourselves

When I think about the one of the most important qualities necessary to be a successful sexologist, courage comes to mind. Courage is necessary when policymakers advocate for change in reproductive healthcare, when educators address stigma surrounding sexuality in the classroom, and when clinicians confront sex-negative societal views with their clients. Surrogate partners, somatic sex educators, and sex workers all need courage to maintain personal safety in their workplace.

In the sexuality business, courage and believing in ourselves is essential. However, for many of us, believing in ourselves is much easier said than done. One of the largest threats to entrepreneurs believing in themselves is imposter syndrome. Identified by psychologists Pauline Clance and Suzanne Imes in 1978, imposter syndrome is phenomenon that occurs when people perceive themselves as inadequate, inferior or not good enough, despite having adequate evidence indicating their accomplishments (Dalla-Camina, 2018). Thus, feeling like an "imposter" in one's own life. Imposter syndrome is not considered a psychological diagnosis, however, it can be comorbid with stress, anxiety, low self-confidence, depression and shame.

Furthermore, imposter syndrome manifests in self-doubt which can be debilitating for business too. When we are new in business and we are making our first hire, there is a lot of room for self-doubt to creep in.

Self-doubt may sound like:

Who would want to work for me?
Why would someone ever work for me?
What if I hire the wrong person?
Others have already done this, better than I ever could. What's the point?

Do any of these thoughts sound familiar? Chances are we have experienced similar doubts in our lifetime. The estimated prevalence of imposter syndrome varies from 9% to 82% with greater symptoms experienced by women (Bravata et al., 2020; Nance-Nash, 2020; Sakulku & Alexander, 2011), women of color (Nance-Nash, 2020), and entrepreneurs (Ladge et al., 2019; Mann, 2019). Women likely experience higher rates of imposter syndrome because of their consistent underrepresentation and lack of support in leadership roles. One study conducted by an independent research firm (that develops global equity indexes) found roughly 20% of directors globally were women (Milhomem, 2020), which means nearly 80% of director positions were held by people other than women. Another study that surveyed over 423 companies found convincing evidence that women of color only account for 4% of C-suite leaders, women in leadership roles are more likely to experience microaggressions, and over half of women leaders who manage teams are almost always burned out (LeanIn.org & McKinsey & Company, 2021). These findings would suggest women (and people on the margin) in leadership positions experience specific challenges based on their identities, which may explain why they are particularly vulnerable to experiencing imposter syndrome and self-doubt. Entrepreneurs commonly experience self-doubt as they are acting in many roles simultaneously and engaging in continuous executive decision-making. Sex-preneurs need to recognize that experiencing doubt is part of the human experience and it absolutely does not disqualify someone from doing this work.

Here is how NOT to get squashed by self-doubt:

1. Create a recognition record.

    One of the biggest ways self-doubt and imposter syndrome take over is by sweeping all our accomplishments under the rug and then complaining about how the rug is dirty and we are not worthy of the rug...and as a mental health professional, I know that avoiding our accomplishments does no one any good. Instead, we need to recognize our accomplishments of all magnitudes. Repeat after me, "Next time I make progress in growing my business, I will record it." Keep a journal (or a digital spreadsheet) with space to recognize each upcoming business move. Made a hiring decision? Record it. Got a new client? Record it. Receive a testimonial? Record it. Next, set up a time each week to review the recognition record and reflect on the evident growth thus far. None of us would be here without each of these moments.

2. Start therapy.

Therapy is one of the best investments one can make in oneself as they are going through this process. Individual therapy also happens to be immensely helpful in addressing symptoms of imposter syndrome like self-doubt (Weir, 2013). Reaching out to a healthcare provider to get referrals for a therapist can be a starting point. Inclusive Therapists, Open Path Psychotherapy Collective, Therapy for Black Girls, and Psychology Today are online directories that connect clients with therapists based on their specialization and zip code.

3. Create an advisory board.

No, this is not the kind of board that meets annually to fundraise for a local non-profit. A personal advisory board are a small hand-selected group of individuals (I recommend no more than four people) who we share a high degree of trust with, are educated about different aspects of business and they know us well and are not afraid to challenge us. Consulting our board of advisors is useful if we find ourselves stuck when making a hiring decision.

4. Remember, self-doubt is normal.

If it is not super clear already, experiencing self-doubt while building a business is incredibly common. Experiencing self-doubt is most certainly not an indication that we are unfit to be on this sex-preneurial journey. Just because we did not get a guidebook for how to hire staff does not mean we are not qualified to do so. Think about the sex-preneurs we all know and admire. Who are they? How did they get to where they are today? Each time we feel self-doubt, we ought to remember they experienced doubts too. And we can still do this work. Learning to manage self-doubt can be instrumental before focusing on our business needs.

Identifying Our Business Needs

Understanding our business needs is essential before beginning the hiring process. In fact, hiring without direction in terms of fit can be counterproductive. For example, if a person manages a therapy practice and has a surplus of client referrals, one may think hiring a therapist who can provide direct service to clients would be what they need. Right? Not exactly. Hiring clinicians who can provide direct service may be the overall goal, but greater information about our ideal candidate is needed to clarify goodness of fit. As sex-preneurs, we need to think critically about who the right fit for our businesses will be, which means understanding the personal and experiential qualities necessary for the role.

Here are some questions sex-preneurs can use to determine their ideal candidate:

- What type of training would this individual already need to have to excel in this role?
- If a candidate does not have as much training, what kind of training is the business able to provide this individual?
- Which interpersonal skills are most vital for this individual to have?
- How does this candidate define sex-positivity and how does their definition align with the company's definition?
- Which personality traits are most important for this person to thrive in our business?
- What personal attributes or skills are less relevant for this role?
- Do they need to be analytical? Organized? Engaging? Team oriented? Passionate?

Our answers to these questions can be helpful in guiding our job description. Ultimately, we want to attract people that are going to see themselves in the job description. Narrow in on skills and attributes that are most essential—separating into required and requested can be a good idea. We also need to make sure the tone of the description also matches the tone of our company. If the soul of our business is wildly energetic, we ought to infuse that energy into the language we use in our application process and materials.

Employers ought to be aware of how employees' personality and work environment play a role when building their team, as supported by theories. Person-Environment Fit theory (Van Vianen, 2018) suggests both the person and environment predict human behavior and outcomes are greater when people's environments align with their own personal needs. Similarly, strengths use theory (Bakker & van Woerkom, 2018) also argues employees fair better if their personality aligns with their work environment. Understanding our employees' personality types can guide our search for finding our next hire. Several studies have explored the relevance of personality type in predicting employee's work engagement and satisfaction (Ghayas et al., 2022; Herr et al., 2021; Murtza et al., 2020). However, I know few sex-preneurs who utilize these tools to help guide their hiring processes because they are quite costly and not the most accessible for small businesses. Without this data, sex-preneurs may not be able to predict how well a new hire will fit in their team.

Using online assessment tools may be helpful particularly if we already have an established business and are approaching expanding. For example, The Predictive Index, Kolbe, and Clifton Strengths are online platforms employers can use to evaluate existing and prospective hires' behavioral patterns and personality traits to determine the best fit for their team. While not every sex-preneur in startup phase will have the resources to use programs like these, understanding employee's personal attributes is important when making hiring decisions.

Replication in Practice

Understanding how to locate, attract, and keep qualified candidates is critical to creating a sustainable and profitable sexuality business. If we have an established business with employees, consider, who are the rockstars (i.e., professionals who excel at their key tasks, are motivated, and work collaboratively with others) on our team already? Identifying the skills and personal qualities they have can help guide our expansion efforts. Essentially, we need to consider, why is this employee such a rockstar? Next, we need to tailor our search to look for candidates with similar skills. This process is called replication. Replication is the process of pinpointing themes, skills, and systems that are functioning well in our business and using that data to find talented individuals who can carry them out. Replication is not designed to create homogeneity in terms of employees' personal demographics, but instead prioritize the most valuable skill and personality traits relevant to specific positions. Replicating is a reliable approach to hiring that teaches employers to use data to drive decision processes for future hires. This data helps employers make more confident hiring decisions.

Finding talent is only half the equation when it comes to hiring. Employers also need to accurately represent their work environment and professional dynamics. The work environment may include aspects of culture, expectations, interpersonal dynamics, management style, and more. Interpersonal relationships in the workplace, including management style, influence employees' job satisfaction (Schuster, 2019). Without conveying an accurate scope of the work environment, job seekers may be reticent to apply or stay engaged in a hiring process.

Self-reflection is a tool that helps us define these important details. As such, I have included some questions to help guide us along the way. The following questions are separated into two categories: internal and external. Internal questions are about the individual and their business as it presents today. External questions are questions that the hiring manager might ask about specific candidates during the interview process.

We can use these questions to understand our business dynamics better:

Internal

- What personality types are going to thrive working alongside the operations manager? (Perhaps this is the owner or another employee)
- How would we describe our management style?
- How do we present feedback? How do we receive feedback?
- As a manager, who would we work well with?
- How would we describe the culture of our business?
- If we are hiring additional people, who are the rock stars of our team already?

External

- Would our style mesh well with ____ type of candidate? Can we adapt to them?
- Will working with this candidate help us grow as a manager?
- Will this candidate bring ____ (important quality) to the team?
- How will this candidate support/engage with the remainder of our team?
- What can our team learn from this candidate?

Solo sex-preneurs who intend to manage new prospective employees for the first time should consider consulting a few people who know them well and ask them to describe their work ethic and management approach. Sex-preneurs who currently have employees that they manage could ask these employees to describe their approach to management. This is a great way to check in on their working relationships and explore any feedback that may be helpful moving forward. Once we have clearly identified our business needs and our business environment, we are ready to examine our values.

Developing A Value-Congruent Process

As sex-preneurs, we tend to have familiarity with showcasing our personal brand and highlighting the unique reasons why clients hire us. A personal brand is a message that conveys an individual's skills, personality, and values to others in an identifiable way (Montoya, 2002). Without our brand awareness and these marketing initiatives, we would not be able to generate paying customers. The same rationale can be applied for prospective employees. Job seekers are eager to understand how the work experience will feel, opportunities for growth, and whether our company values align with them. Candidates are seeking information that extends beyond the job responsibilities which ultimately drives their decision of whether to apply.

In an era focused on social responsibility, more and more job seekers are paying attention to a company's values and mission. This is aligned with research discussing how values play a significant role in the occupational choices people make and can predict their behaviors and decisions (Arieli et al., 2020; Bustamante et al., 2021). A few studies have found Millennial job seekers are placing more importance on aspects of the company (e.g., a company's values/mission, work culture, level of flexibility, etc.) they work for instead of the material factors such as compensation (Ng et al., 2010; Ismail & Lu, 2014). Other research suggests job seekers are more attracted to employers with similar values to their own (Cable & Judge, 1996). Businesses cannot be exempt from showcasing their values—without such visibility, they will run the risk of economic rupture from inability to hire qualified candidates.

What does this mean for us as sex-preneurs?

Our values need to be accessible for job seekers and they need to inform every aspect of our business, including the hiring process. This means that our values are not just visible to applicants and our clientele, but these values ought to inform the decisions we are making internally. For example, if accountability is one of our company's values, how is that reflected in our work culture and leadership? Perhaps we have a process where employees can evaluate their leaders from which leaders address and are held accountable to make changes in their work environment. To promote safety in this process, employees could share feedback anonymously and leaders ought to be responsive to feedback shared by creating a specific action plan that is tailored to feedback shared. Employees and leaders could each nominate supplementary individuals outside the organization to report to during this accountability process (i.e., by considering complaints or conducting leadership reviews). Ensuring alignment between company values and plans for evaluation, growth, and reporting complaints is a useful practice for sex-preneurs.

Too often, businesses have named their values externally without any alignment internally. A company that claims to value accountability but lacks a clear accountability structure for their staff to engage in when harm happens has a value incongruency. This incongruency could suggest the business either needs support on how to develop value aligned structures or the process of naming their values is motivated by social desirability and is only meant to benefit them. Naming values externally without alignment internally is perceived as disingenuous and impersonal. Some scholars have referred to this phenomenon as "performative" or "performative allyship" (Kalina, 2020; McKellar, 2021). As sex-preneurs, value alignment is critical given the scope of work we provide. Therefore, if we are going to do the work to define our company values, what is the point of doing that work if it does not inform our business practices?

We can use these questions to reflect on our business values:

- What are the values of our business?
- How are our values apparent to prospective applicants? How are our values evident to our clients/consumers?
- How do we uphold these values in our business?
- How are our values evident throughout the application process?
- Are our values congruent with our business practices and policies? If not, which practices/policies need to shift?

As we reflect and actively assess our alignment of our business' values, we may have clarity about areas of growth that are needed. Documenting ideas in a chart can be helpful to keep track of each value, policy, and alignment status, like this one here:

Value	Policy	Alignment?

After we have critically examined our values and business practices, we are ready to think critically about how to adapt our policies and procedures to be more in alignment with our values. Since developing and implementing these changes can be a large undertaking for many business owners, engaging a consultant who specializes in alignment work and business policy development can be a worthwhile decision. While most of these referrals tend to be generated by word of mouth, there are a few organizations I can personally recommend. Praxis Group is a group of consultants who specialize in helping businesses redefine group and organizational cultures and create more alignment with their values. Jesse Holzman is a sociologist and consultant who helps businesses develop accountability structures (for performance and evaluation) in addition to transparent reporting processes that center restorative practices. Social media can be another way to connect with consultants and organizational business professionals. Social media is also a vehicle that job seekers may use to assess a company's values based on their media presence. In the next chapter, we will explore the relevance of media and promotion.

Embracing the Art of Shameless Self-Promotion

One of the most common questions I hear from business owners about hiring is, where am I finding candidates? This is a pertinent question, particularly during times when the job market has been slow or oversaturated. Historically, hiring and retaining skillful employees has been one of the most difficult tasks for employers and leaders of global organizations (Bilan et al., 2020; Krishnan & Scullion, 2017). Possible explanations for why employers tend to have a difficult time filling vacancies include a shortage of employees with necessary skills, factors impacting the attractiveness of the market (e.g., pay, benefits, hours), inefficient recruitment procedures, and job satisfaction (Bilan et al., 2020). Sex-preneurs need a savvy approach to hiring to withstand these challenges. While existing research on talent management is not specific to sexuality businesses, one could argue hiring may be more challenging for sex-preneurs given our niche industry. If we are hiring a sexuality consultant, we are probably looking for candidates who already have training in human sexuality and hold an advanced degree in counseling or organizational psychology. This individual is going to likely require more lead time than if we are looking to fill an administrative role because the necessary skills and qualifications apply to a broader group. Maintaining realistic expectations based on the conditions of the current job market and having patience is important when beginning a search.

Getting the word out about job postings has certainly changed over the years with the advancement of technology. Utilizing sexology listservs, social media accounts (e.g., Instagram, LinkedIn, Twitter, and Facebook) and generating e-newsletters are modern electronic marketing initiatives that many job seekers use (Subbarao et al., 2022). Presenting at conferences, getting our work published and establishing relationships with other sex-ologists are additional recommendations for promotion (Taverner, 2006). As sex-preneurs, we ought to make savvy, research-based decisions about where and how we promote open positions so we can reach the candidates we are looking for.

Determining which avenues to use for promotion is important to be financially and energetically efficient. While some people have found suc-cess utilizing job search ads or directories, I have not found those to be most effective in generating applicants who are aligned with our mission and scope of work. I have found job search websites to be effective at generat-ing a large quantity of applicants and accessing candidates who we may not otherwise be able to reach due to location and network. Many job search websites require a fee for service to boost reach, so sex-preneurs should be prepared to budget accordingly if planning to utilize this method for their search. Altogether, I think the utility of job search websites depends on the specific role a business is looking to fill and the breath of applicants' neces-sary qualifications.

There are many routes to finding the right applicant. Indicating key prac-tical and interpersonal skills needed for the role can be helpful during mar-keting the position because it can help others identify who a good fit may be. Key practical skills I look for include excellent verbal and nonverbal communication, attending to and reflecting emotions, active listening, lead-ing/directing others, and problem management. Interpersonal skills I look for in a hire include strong communication and listening skills (i.e., con-veying information clearly, giving and receiving feedback well), empathy, curiosity and willingness to learn, warmth, a collaborative approach, and a positive attitude. In my experience, I have found personal referrals provide the best recommendations because they know me and my business well. When I am hiring, I send email blasts to my professional networks, include an announcement in my company's monthly newsletter, post frequently on our social media accounts, and bring up our hiring needs in conversation with my friends and colleagues. This is where the significance of shameless self-promotion comes in.

When sex-preneurs are hiring, we must get comfortable with broadcast-ing our needs to the world. This can be particularly challenging for peo-ple who are used to maintaining a lot of privacy, people who are more introverted, or people who have anxious thoughts about putting themselves out there. For example, some of us do not use social media much and the thought of putting ourselves out there on LinkedIn might feel like a massive leap…and that is understandable. Embracing self-promotion is likely to feel uncomfortable at first and it can have a massive return on our businesses. Remember, growing a business means growing ourselves! So, I recommend normalizing the sh** out of that discomfort. Additionally, exposure activities can help people build confidence with self-promotion.

Sex-preneurs can practice self-promotion by:

- Casually mentioning something they are working on in their business to a personal services provider (e.g., chiropractor, barber/hair stylist, physical therapist, esthetician, massage therapist, scuba instructor, personal trainer, nail technician).
- Engaging with likeminded companies and professionals on social media.
- Informing a colleague they are thinking about hiring at a meet-and-greet event.
- Asking if anyone has any leads for their position at a consultation group meeting.
- Consulting with a trusted sex-preneur about their hiring process.
- Announcing they are hiring to their friends while hanging out.
- Introducing their business to their neighbors at a block party.
- Highlighting new business offerings at their local chamber of commerce networking event.

As with most things, the more experience we have with self-promotion, the less daunting it tends to feel. Confidence cannot grow without discomfort. Yes, putting our businesses out into the world is vulnerable and can feel uneasy, and I promise it is also 100% worth it.

Following Our Intuition

There is no secret sauce when it comes to growing a business, however, there are a few precious gems that every sex-preneur should know. These lessons I have learned throughout my own sex-preneurial journey, and I hope they can add value for others' too.

1. Attend to our intuition and engage in reflective thinking:

    Intuition has consistently been declared as an important factor in decision making and entrepreneurial cognition (Armstrong & Hird, 2009; Baldacchino, 2019; Bohm & Brun, 2008; Gillin et al., 2018; Soosalu et al., 2019), though limited to few empirical studies exist to confirm these assertions. One study found associations between individuals' preferences for intuition and having more positive attitudes toward entrepreneurship and entrepreneurship intentions (Castellano et al., 2014). Other anecdotal information suggests intuition is a vital skill for entrepreneurs, which I think is highly relevant despite the limited convincing evidence available.

Curating a team with intention means considering applicants' knowledge, skills, personality, and ethos during the interview process and attending to visceral feelings in addition to practical assessments when evaluating goodness of fit. Our emotions, gut feelings, intuition, and reasoning shape our information processing (Haidt, 2013), which can be highly relevant when hiring employees. Therefore, listening to our intuition during the hiring process is essential. Hiring decisions are some of the most significant and costly decisions sex-preneurs can make. When we hire someone to join our team, we are inviting them to both perform a set of duties (their job) and to represent our brand. Employees' behavior reflects the culture and reputation of a company, which is instrumental to our success. As employers, we must realize that we sometimes have limited information to go from during the hiring process before extending an offer of employment. While employers can amend an employment agreement should an employee not work out, onboarding new employees can be expensive. Thus, paying attention to intuitive responses during the interview process is important.

2. Create space for processing:

As sex-preneurs, we are often extremely busy with packed schedules. Especially in the beginning, we are juggling it all—financial decisions, taxes, marketing initiatives, content/product development, payroll, etc. This means that at any given moment we are likely to have many tabs open in our minds, which can present as distraction from the current moment and leave us vulnerable to miss important details. I have found it helpful to block off time before and after interviews to process the interactions. Before the interview, I use the time to transition from one task to another and to reflect on topics I want to cover with an applicant. I have found that even five minutes of buffer time has made a huge impact in how present I feel during interviews. After the interview, I key into how I am feeling in my body, think about any outstanding questions I have, note what I was drawn to about the candidate, and highlight any reservations. During this time, I am checking in with various domains: my head, my heart, and my gut.

3. Consult with a trusted source:

Once I have processed independently, I find it incredibly valuable to process with my team. When I am in conversation with my team about a candidate, I tend to become more aware of my feelings about the process overall. My team knows me well at this point, so they tend to mirror my energy back towards me. If I am feeling unsure about a candidate, they will point that out and share their own experiences. They are familiar with company culture enough to know which qualities to assess goodness of fit and who would complement our team. Since many sex-preneurs do not have a team when they start out, this would be a great time to consult one's board of directors.

Once I have gone through each of these stages, I reassess. Do I feel clearer on a path forward? If I am not certain about a candidate, I will not move forward.

This is one of the biggest lessons I have learned thus far. I would much rather hire a candidate who I confidently feel is a great fit than hire one that I am unclear about. There were times when I did not fully trust my gut, consult with my team or leave space for processing—and I know I learned from them the hard way. During these times, I recognized wavering gut feelings internally and I decided to prioritize others' assessments over my own intuition, which lead to turmoil. Learning to prioritize gut feelings has been an instrumental lesson in my sex-preneurial journey that I hope others can learn from too.

Conclusion

Growing a business is an exciting moment filled with great privilege and responsibilities. The people we hire can have a substantial impact on the direction of our growth. Without strong hires, businesses are unable to provide the same caliber of services or products, which can negatively impact their reputation and overall revenue generation. In this industry, people are one of the most important factors to a successful business, further emphasizing the need for quality hires. Quality hires tend to be driven to employers based on compensation, benefits, flexibility, growth opportunities, value alignment, and culture. Creating positions that keenly cater to job seekers' interests is a useful strategy for sex-preneurs. To engage in effective hiring, sex-preneurs also need to maintain a growth-oriented mindset, clearly identify their business needs, develop value-congruent processes, embrace self-promotion, and follow their intuition. Recognizing when to reach out for help (e.g., engaging a consultant or coach) and building community with trustworthy other sex-preneurs can help enhance confidence throughout the process. While sex-preneurs may not receive a roadmap for hiring in business, we have a lot we can learn from one another along the way.

Questions for Reflection

- What is preventing you from creating a profitable and sustainable business?

- What are the top three hiring-related challenges you faced in your business in the last 12 months? How did you navigate them? What did you learn from these challenges?

- On a scale of one to five, how does your business align with your values? Name three specific examples for each value.

- Which practices are serving your business well? What are you most proud of?

- What kind of business support would be most valuable for you right now?

- What piece of advice would you give yourself (a week/month/year) ago now that you are where you are today?

References

Arieli, S., Sagiv, L., & Roccas, S. (2020). Values at work: The impact of personal values in organisations. *Applied Psychology*, 69(2), 230–275. doi: 10.1111/apps.12181

Armstrong, S., & Hird, A. (2009). Cognitive style and entrepreneurship drive of new and mature business owners-managers. *Journal of Business Psychology*, 24, 419–430. https://doi.org/10.1007/s10869-009-9114-4

Baldacchino, L. (2019). Intuition in entrepreneurial cognition. In: Caputo, A., & Pellegrini, M. (eds)., *The anatomy of entrepreneurial decisions. Contributions to management science*. Springer. https://doi.org/10.1007/978-3-030-19685-1_3

Bakker, A. B., & van Woerkom, M. (2018). Strengths use in organizations: A positive approach of occupational health. *Canadian Psychology/Psychologie Canadienne*, 59(1), 38–46. https://doi.org/10.1037/cap0000120.

Bilan, Y., Mishchuk, H., Roshchyk, I., & Joshi, O. (2020). Hiring and retaining skilled employees in SMEs: Problems in human resource practices and links with organizational success. *Business: Theory and Practice*, 21(2), 780–791. https://doi.org/10.3846/btp.2020.12750

Bohm, G., & Brun, W. (2008). Intuition and affect in risk perception and decision making. *Judgment and Decision Making*, 3, 1–4.

Bravata, D. M., Madhusudhan, D. K., Boroff, M., & Cokley, K. O. (2020). Commentary: Prevalence, predictors, and treatment of imposter syndrome: A systematic review. *Journal of Mental Health and Clinical Psychology*, 4(3), 12–16. https://doi.org/10.29245/2578-2959/2020/3.1207

Bustamante, S., Ehlscheidt, R., Pelzeter, A., Deckmann, A., & Freudenberger, F. (2021). The effect of values on the attractiveness of responsible employers for young job seekers. *Journal of Human Values*, 27(1), 27–48. https://doi.org/10.1177/0971685820973522

Cable, D. M., Judge, T. A. (1996). Person–organization fit, job choice decisions, and organizational entry. *Organizational Behavior and Human Decision Processes*, 67(3), 294–311.

Castellano, S., Maalaoui, A., Safraou, I., & Reymond, E. (2014). Linking intuition and entrepreneurial intention: A comparative study among French and US student entrepreneurs. *International Journal of Entrepreneurship and Innovation Management*, 18(1), 23–44.

Certification types: Distinguishing sexuality educators, counselors, and therapists. (2022). Retrieved July 13, 2022, from https://www.aasect.org/certification-types -distinguishing-sexuality-educators-counselors-and-therapists

Dalla-Camina, M. The reality of imposter syndrome. *Psychology Today*, September 3, 2018. https://www.psychologytoday.com/us/blog/real-women/201809/the -reality-imposter-syndrome

Freire, I. (2018, August 2). Interview with Luis Perelman. Sociedade Portuegesa de Sexologia Clínica. https://spsc.pt/index.php/2018/08/02/in-most-countries -sexologists-have-not-been-as-political-as-they-should/

Ghayas, M. M., Shaheen, A., & Devi, A. (2022). Personality, job satisfaction and organizational commitment. *Reviews of Management Sciences*, 3(2), 101–113. https://doi.org/10.53909/admin.v3i2.100

Gillin, L. M., Gagliardi, R. Hougaz, L., Knowles, D., & Langhammer, M. (2018). Teaching companies how to be entrepreneurial: Cultural change at all levels, *Journal of Business Strategy*, 40(2), 59–67. https://doi.org/10.1108/JBS-09-2017-0138

Haidt, J. (2013). *The righteous mind*. Vintage Books, Division of Random House, New York.

Herr, R. M., van Vianen, A. E. M., Bosle, C., & Fischer, J. E. (2021). Personality type matters: Perceptions of job demands, job resources, and their associations with work engagement and mental health. *Current Psychology*. https://doi.org/10.1007/s12144-021-01517-w

Ismail, M., & Lu, H. S. (2014). Cultural values and career goals of the millennial generation: An integrated conceptual framework. *The Journal of International Management Studies*, 9(1), 38–49.

Kalina, P. (2020). Performative allyship. *Technium Social Sciences Journal*, 11(1), 478–481.

Krishnan, T. N., & Scullion, H. (2017). Talent management and dynamic view of talent in small and medium enterprises. *Human Resource Management Review*, 27(3), 431–441. https://doi.org/10.1016/j.hrmr.2016.10.003

Ladge, J., Eddleston, K. A., & Sugiyama, K. (2019). Am I an entrepreneur? How imposter fears hinder women entrepreneurs' business growth. *Business Horizons*, 62(5), 615–624. https://doi.org/10.1016/j.bushor.2019.05.001.

Lazkani, S. (2021, March 12). Lebanese stand behind sexologist who was bullied during a TV interview. *Lebanon News*. https://www.the961.com/lebanese-stand-behind-sexologist-atallah/

LeanIn.org, & McKinsey & Company. (2021). *Women in the workplace*. https://wiw-report.s3.amazonaws.com/Women_in_the_Workplace_2021.pdf

Levand, M. A., & Canan, S. N. (2018). Navigating sexualization as a sexuality professional: Recommendations from sexuality educators at the 2016 National Sex Ed Conference. *American Journal of Sexuality Education*, 13(1), 94–107. https://doi.org/10.1080/15546128.2018.1433566

Mann, S. (2019). *Why do I feel like an imposter? How to understand and cope with imposter syndrome*. Watkins Media Limited.

McKellar, E. (2021). *Shopping for a cause: Social influencers, performative allyship, and the commodification of activism* [Unpublished master's thesis]. California State University San Bernadino.

Milhomem, C. (2020). Women on boards: 2020 progress report. MSCI.

Montoya, P. (2002). *The personal branding phenomenon*. Personal Branding Press.

Murtza, M. H., Gill, S. A., Aslam, H. D,, & Noor, A. (2020). Intelligence quotient, job satisfaction, and job performance: The moderating role of personality type. *Journal of Public Affairs*, 21(3), e2318. https://doi.org/10.1002/pa.2318

Nance-Nash, S. (2020, July 27). Why imposter syndrome hits women and women of colour harder. *Equality Matters*. https://www.bbc.com/worklife/article/20200724-why-imposter-syndrome-hits-women-and-women-of-colour-harder

Ng, E. S. W., Schweitzer, L., & Lyons, S. T. (2010). New generation, great expectations. A field study of the millennial generation. *Journal of Business and Psychology*, 25, 281–292.

Pillai-Friedman, S., Pollitt, J. L. & Castaldo, A. (2014). Becoming kink-aware – A necessity for sexuality professionals. *Sexual and Relationship Therapy*, 30(2), 196–210. https://doi.org/10.1080/14681994.2014.975681

Roach, M. (2008). *Bonk: The curious coupling of science and sex*. W.W. Norton & Company, Inc.

Sakulku, J., & Alexander, J. (2011). The imposter phenomenon. *International Journal of Behavioral Science*, 6(1), 75–97. https://doi.org/10.14456/ijbs.2011.6

Schuster, E. (2019, April 19). *Indiana University*. Who's the Boss? The Role of Management Style and Communication in the Workplace. Retrieved May 18, 2022, from https://scholarworks.iu.edu/dspace/handle/2022/23027

Soosalu, G., Henwood, S., & Deo, A. (2019). Head, heart, and gut in decision making: Development of a multiple brain preference questionnaire. *SAGE Open*. https://doi.org/10.1177/2158244019837439

Sri Kantha, S. (2021). Sexology of Wardell Pomeroy: An analysis. *International Medical Journal*, *28*(6), 667–670. https://www.researchgate.net/publication /357331343_Sexography_of_Wardell_Pomeroy_Int_Med_J_Dec_2021_286 _667-670

Subbarao, N.V., Chhabra, B., & Mishra, M. (2022). Social media usage behavior in job search: Implications for corporate image and employer branding. In: Rajagopal & R. Behl (eds.) *Managing disruptions in business. Palgrave Studies in Democracy, Innovation, and Entrepreneurship for Growth* (pp. 51–79). London, United Kingdom: Palgrave Macmillan Cham. https://doi.org/10.1007/978-3-030 -79709-6_3

Tiefer, L. (1994). Three crises facing sexology. *Archives of Sexual Behavior*, *23*(4), 361–374.

Taverner, W. J. (2006). Tips for emerging sexology professionals: Networking and nurturing. *Contemporary Sexuality*.

Van Vianen, A. E. (2018). Person–environment fit: A review of its basic tenets. *Annual Review of Organizational Psychology and Organizational Behavior*, *5*(1), 75–101. https://doi.org/10.1146/annurev-orgpsych-032117-104702.

Weir, K. (November 2013). "Feel like a fraud?" *grad PSYCH Magazine*, *11*(4). https://www.apa.org/gradpsych/2013/11/fraud#:~:text=For%20many %20people%20with%20impostor,to%20fly%20under%20the%20radar.

4 Navigating Touch

Ethics and Triadic Relationships

Fredrick Zal

Introduction

A client might hold depression, chronic pelvic pain, or have relationship turmoil when they employ a "Sexpert"; but the client is looking for assistance specifically around the topics of sex. Sexual healthcare providers need the skills and practice to effectively role-model navigating sexual attraction, expectations, boundaries, and consensual touch in the safety of the consultation room. Role-modeling can support healthcare without harmful perpetuation of sexual shame, stigma, and marginalization. Evidence-based clinical practices have assisted clients in the creation of more joy and less harm in nuanced sexual complexity from the streets to the sheets.

This writing engages the lived experiences of intimate sensuality/sexuality interpersonal dynamics and touch experiences to focus the complexity of defining sexual behavior (Plummer, 1975) and sexualization (Gagnon & Simon, 1973). Haptic skill-building techniques and empathic approaches are proposed for inclusion in professional practice, or referral to another sexuality professional to support the importance of touch and interpersonal connections for clients, both solo and in relationships. These techniques require metacognition of values, boundaries, and limitations concurrently personal and professional. The practice of these techniques by the reader, or a sexuality professional, assists in the critical and transformational cognitive-somatic processing of both the client and the professional. Exploitation, coercion, harming, and/or influencing a client away from self-determination are completely unacceptable! Recommendations assist professionals to avoid pitfalls, heal multicultural sensual/sexual erasure, and strategically plan businesses for professional collaborations with a range of disciplines. To foster connective sexuality healthcare; services are intended to be client-centered, role model incremental risk processing, vulnerability, and love.

Care service providers that might refer sensuality and sexuality clients range from activists, advocates, aromatherapy, beauty work, chefs, child care, clergy, dentists, esthetician, fashion designers, first responders (fire, police, paramedics, etc.), hair stylists, health aides, hygienists, photographers,

DOI: 10.4324/9781003314660-4

physician assistants, policy makers, researchers, tattoo artists, undertakers, and other paraprofessionals in a spectrum of disciplines. Additionally, due to the body-focused work of acupuncturists, alternative medicine, massage therapists, nurses, physicians from diverse specialties, and yoga teachers there is the potential to bump up against the boundaries of professional services and eroticism. Professionals who are trained academically or through apprentice traditions to assist in lifespan sexuality development are coaches, counselors, escorts, physiotherapists, professional dominants, prostitutes, psychiatrists, psychologists, reflexologists, school counselors, sex workers, sexologists, sexuality educators, shamanic healers, social workers, somatic bodyworkers, strippers, surrogates, tantrika, and therapists. Within this diverse range of professional traditions, there is very little agreement upon how to professionally engage sexuality.

Alfred Kinsey, Betty Dodson, Caffyn Jesse, Ted McIlvenna, Victoria Johnson, Wilhelm Reich, and other sexologists have all implored that the sexuality professions recognize people are "pumping fleshy biological creatures who heave and hump, sweat and slide, and deliver orgasmic frenzies" (Plummer, 2012). "Ironically, the vast majority of sexuality research, [education, and therapy] does not have much sex in it" (Tolman, 2014). Euro-American culture is saturated with a McDonaldized folie à deux (shared delusion) of erotic desire through highly sexualized visual, text, and auditory media (Baudrillard, 1981, 90; Foucault, 1978, 58; Fine & McClelland, 2006; MacFarlane, Fuller, Wakefield, & Brents, 2017). Yet, due to a long legacy of genuine sensual embodiment beyond the mechanics of procreation being highly taboo (Rubin, 1984; 2011); many have grown-up sexually foreclosed (Marcia, 1966). Some people do not have a sense of sensual/sexual self, knowing what they differently desire each day, what they have to offer another, nor how to navigate the interpersonal complexity of sex. A false sense of connection brought with virtual social media and approximately two years of COVID-19 isolation has widened this sensual/sexual disconnect. Therefore, the global population is at a time when creating genuine relationships and sharing consensual touch can be especially healing.

Affirmative sensuality will assist in healing this cultural foreclosure and disconnection. Sex positivity is a community of people who "don't denigrate, medicalize, or demonize any form of sexual expression except that which is not consensual" (Queen, 1997, 128). Barker and Jane (2016, 390) further define sex positivism to believe that sexual freedom is an inalienable right, while acknowledging that currently only a privileged few can access it. Emotional connection and physical pleasure are legitimate and ethically integral to life. Sex positivity does not imply sexual access, desire, nor sexual behavior quantities. Being sex positive means that one's approach to sensuality / sexuality has a comfort and ease, be that in words or touch. Sex positivity is not about the quantity of sexual interpersonal nor solo masturbatory engagements. Therefore, one can as easily be asexual, celibate, or a nymphomaniac, and all be sex positive. Re-claiming sex positivism will re-inform our bodies to transcend hegemonic socio-cultural rhetoric (Kennedy & Dean, 1995, 20-21), to re-eroticize the de-eroticized capitalist body (Williams & Bendelow, 1998, 105), and thereby release all people from tyranny.

Ethic Codes for Sexuality Healthcare Service Providers

The codification of "appropriate" sexuality in 21 professional healthcare service provider policies in the United States and Britain are examined. The American Medical Association (AMA) was founded in 1847 as the world built upon the foundations of the Euro-American Industrial Revolution (1760–1840). It was a time that focused upon urbanized ideals of productivity, workers, and purging of ancestral land-based physical, emotional, and spiritual connections. Nearly 12 million people, primarily from England, Ireland, and Germany had fled oppression or seized dreams of "opportunity" to further colonize what is now called the United States between 1870 and 1900. With these mostly Anglo-Saxon immigrants came the societal ideals of Freud, von Krafft-Ebing, and the founding of the American Psychological Association (APA) in 1892. Soon followed by the formation of the American Nursing Association (ANA) in 1896 and the American Osteopathic Association (AOA) in 1897. These four private biomedical organizations had created the basis for all modern sexological ethics. The American Association of Naturopathic Physicians (AANP) was recently founded in 1985, in support of the American College of Traditional Chinese Medicine's first class of graduating students. The American Traditional Chinese Medicine Association (ATCMA), registered in 2016, does not have a publicly available code of ethics. Modern binary-gendered reproductive medicine was institutionalized through the American Urological Association and the American College of Obstetricians and Gynecologists. Policy from the American Association for Marriage and Family Therapy (AAMFT); American Association of Sexuality Educators Counselors and Therapists (AASECT); American Counseling Association (ACA); National Association of Social Workers (NASW); and Therapist Certification Association (TCA) was also reviewed in this chapter's analysis. The British Association for Counselling and Psychotherapy (BACP) policy has been compared for a cross-Atlantic perspective.

The moral philosophies in the codes of ethics are clearly based upon the lineages of modern thought coming from Aristotle and Plato (c.330BCE), plus Hume (1740) and Kant (1785; 1788; 1797). The works of Kohlberg (1983), Kitchener (1984; 1996), Punzo and Meara (1993), and Urofsky, Engels, and Engebretson (2008) were informed by Piaget (1932) and Habermas (1990). However, all of the codes and critiques recursively build upon the framework of ethics composed by Beauchamp and Childress (1979; 2019). Much more than the colloquial pastiche of "primum non nocere" (first, do no harm); Beauchamp and Childress (2019) define five focal virtues: compassion, discernment, trustworthiness, integrity, and conscientiousness. These have led to a series of principles that are seen in most all of the professional organizations' codes of ethics: respect for autonomy, nonmaleficence, beneficence, and justice. Professional–patient relationships are strengthened through veracity, privacy, confidentiality, and fidelity. Interpersonal dynamics and bodily experiences in the professional care services provided are cautioned regularly against dual relationships, touch, implied and overt sexuality (Gottlieb, 1993).

Discussion

Of the upmost importance is to differentiate between nonmaleficence and beneficence. "Primum non nocere" (first, do no harm) is an inappropriate translation into Latin from the Hippocratic treatise in Greek: φελέειν ή μ βλάπτειν (oféléein í mí vláptein), which actually means "in illnesses one should keep two things in mind: to be useful, rather than cause no harm" (Retsas, 2019). Within the insurance governed medical-prison-industrial complex; fear mongering is logical to focus away from litigious risk and the potential of harm creation. Beauchamp and Childress (2019, 117) simply state that nonmaleficence can be defined as "one ought not to inflict evil or harm" and that beneficence is more nuanced and empowering in that "one ought to prevent evil or harm… remove evil or harm. [and] do or promote good". "Keeping out of trouble" does not necessitate that one is "doing good" for the client's sexual wellness treatment plan (Brown & Newman, 1992). The American Nursing Association and American Counseling Association support a proactive social justice stance in their policies (ACA, 2014, 8.C; ANA, 2015, vii). The ACA expects professionals to advocate and promote social change for individuals and groups on both institutional and societal levels (2014, 8.C). Professional actions are to remove systemic barriers and obstacles that inhibit client access or provision of appropriate services to improve the quality of life, growth, and development (ACA, 2014, 5; 8.C). The ANA understands that "the lived experiences of inequality, poverty, and social marginalization contribute to the deterioration of health globally" (ANA, 2015, 8.2). Social justice can be augmented through collaboration with other sexuality health professionals as a powerful instrument for change. Sexological professionals, more than any other sector, need to balance their sense of prudery, to "act courageously, and take risks" to help clients (Redlich; in Masters & Johnson, 1977, 148).

An area of significant potential harm perpetuation surrounds the way that autonomy is honored or erased via moral agency. Autonomy can be defined as everyone's intrinsic right to decide what is best for their own mind, body, spirit, story, information, and property for a specific duration of time (Zal, 2019). Generally speaking, this civil right is promoted and upheld with the intent of all of the codes. The ANA is exemplary in stating that all relevant persons (client, care providers, lovers, relatives, etc.) are agentic in the informed decisions for client care (2015, 2.3). The American Medical Association's (AMA) parallel discussion of the physician's exercise of conscience; starts off positively; in that physicians are to respect client's self-determination (AMA, 2022, 1.1.7). However, then the AMA's hubris quickly goes to hell in a handbasket of moral superiority:

> Physicians are not defined solely by their profession. They are moral agents in their own right and, like their patients, are informed by and committed to diverse cultural, religious, and philosophical traditions and beliefs. For some physicians, their professional calling is imbued with their foundational beliefs as persons, and at times the expectation that physicians will put patients' needs and preferences first may be in tension with the need to sustain moral integrity and continuity across both personal and professional life. Preserving opportunity for physicians to act (or to refrain from acting) in accordance with the dictates of conscience in their professional practice is important for preserving the integrity of the medical profession as well as the integrity of the individual physician… physicians should have considerable latitude to practice in accord with well-considered, deeply held beliefs that are central to their self-identities… physicians may be able to act (or refrain from acting) in accordance with the dictates of their conscience without violating their professional obligations… Thoughtfully consider whether and how significantly an action (or declining to act) will undermine the physician's personal integrity, create emotional or moral distress for the physician.
>
> (AMA, 2022, 1.1.7)

This moral superiority has been the justification for the obliteration of client autonomy in a countless number of cases for over a century. If the massiveness of potential harm perpetuation in this policy is not apparent; allow McIlvenna to

> make one thing clear; no matter how smart you are, how wealthy you have become, how many years you went to school, nor how many credentials you have, my body does not belong to you. My body belongs to me.
>
> (1977, 24)

Most contemporary moral philosophers will state that acting from a place of unyielding moral superiority has the great potential of leading to immoral acts (Kitchener, 1984). Yet, this tone of placing the practitioner first, and protecting "the profession" above following client self-determination bleeds through most every code of ethics. The ANA code was built upon the Nightingale Pledge (1935; in ANA, 2015, 47), which vowed loyal subservience to the physician's work. The legacy of physicians' moral agency over "others" has caused such massive abuse, misogyny, invalidation, and sexual harassment that a significant portion of the ANA code is about protecting the civil rights of nurses from colleagues. It is important to also recognize that the hegemonic construction of performative masculinity and assumptions of toxic predatory behavior can also foreclose male bodies from exploration of healthy forms of relatedness and access to bodies without expectations (Twigg, 2011).

To move from a place of potential harmful narcissism, metacognition is very important. This is a process where one's "diverse cultural, religious, and philosophical traditions and beliefs" (AMA, 2022, 1.1.7) are brought to consciousness for reflection and pause. Professional training programs often utilize "dilemmas" specifically because there is zero "one true way" (Jordan, 1990, 109; Barnett, 2007; Jones, et al., 2009), and the nuanced deliberation is informed by differing individual value systems. Both Yarber and Sayad (2010) and the Our Whole Lives (UUA, 2021) curriculum state that it is important to not be "value-free." Understanding the values that one considers to be central to their way of being, these values form a behavioral code (Yarber & Sayad, 2010) to navigate challenging personal decision. Personal values transform into a sense of morality, when one ego-centrically believes that their personal value opinions are applicable to any other person. Societal ethics are created when an elitist group of people sharing a system of values agree in belief that all people should act (or not) in certain ways. This belief is myopic, regardless of what people outside of the hegemonic group believe. These group value systems of ethics are sometimes codified into organizational policies or governmental laws. Professional decisions are to help guide, but not coerce, clients. If professionals cannot hold that line, if professionals center their own values and sense of morality over those of their clients, then they are almost guaranteed to create harm. Reacting in panic and fear to the "chimeras and signifiers" (Rubin, 1984, 297) of false self-centeredness or societal mores rarely alleviates the client's suffering. Sharing of personal values should only be done without expectation to coerce nor influence client self-determination.

Due to centuries of abuse, many marginalized people and groups in society have been pushed too far, and are no longer willing to go along with hegemonic society's pressures and coercion. The #MeToo movement has been strengthening society's appreciation of autonomy, self-determination, and consent. Consent can be defined as an autonomy-focused explicit agreement that mutually respects the boundaries of all people involved, mutual and clear understanding of all information, with no power dynamic influences upon capacity or agency (Zal, 2019). However, Thwaites (2017) strongly warns that focusing on the delusion of autonomous choice in a highly toxic society of power inequity places people at great peril. First, capacity is assumed, unless one is "incapacitated," such as being passed-out drunk on the floor. One-hundred-percent capacity is a cultural myth that might only exist for the first few minutes of the day, after a good night's sleep, having eaten well, and lived in a fulfilling manner the day before. Within moments, our capacity begins to diminish due to substances, physical or emotional exhaustion, arousal or trauma activation, depression, anxiety, and neural diversity. H.A.L.T.S. is a mnemonic to help remember how being hungry or horny, angry, lonely, tired, sick or stressed can diminish capacity. Thwaites (2017) criticizes the flag-bearing of autonomy and choice as a comforting delusion, which placates people to falsely feel empowered and agentic. This veil of comfort stops people from deeply interrogating society. It mires people in a place of "unthinkingness" (ibid.) and acceptance of the existing systems, norms, and tradition. This makes people unaware that seemingly "free choice" is actually foreclosed. "Neoliberal rhetoric of 'choice' is often invested in maintaining the status quo by removing the agency of the less powerful and enhancing that of the established powerful elite" (ibid.). Client autonomy was not in the Hippocratic Oath, early versions of the AMA's policy, nor ancient Chinese medicine simply because clients are always in a place of lowered capacity; since they are approaching care providers in a place of concern for their dis-ease (Tsai, 1999). Add to this the high level of toxicity and personally or vicariously experienced violence (Butler, 2004), all people have diminished capacity. Jesse urges sexologists to assume sexuality clients "do not have ready access to choose and voice around sex" (2020, 23). Power inequity is further skewed if a client is emotionally or physically exposed, weakened, or subject to the surveillance or control of "Sexperts" (Twigg, 2011). For example: a client who is feeling lonely or ill potentially has lowered capacity for autonomous decision making. So, when a "Sexpert" provides a suggestion, the client's decision process is less agentic, and a client might agree with what the professional proposes, even if they would not do such when at full capacity.

Having just experienced two years of COVID isolation and societal panic allows many people to begin comprehending the utter incapacitation of society during the Black Death, which annihilated approximately 50% of Indo-European people between 1348and 1352. Survivors remained in perpetual fear for the next few hundred years. Major epidemics occurred in the late 17th century and recurred regularly until the 19th century, prompting people to panic into "scientific" control of death. During this time, women were the primary healers; midwives that brought their centuries of healing knowledge "from neighbor to neighbor and mother to daughter. They were called 'wise women' by the people, witches or charlatans by the authorities" (Ehrenreich & English, 2010, 25). The transmission of illness was not understood, and these wise women have been targeted by society's fear. Women who were at the heart of society and were loved, cherished, and revered became marginalized and considered as "Other." "In the most ancient mythologies, one finds the expression of a duality; that of the Self and the Other" (De Beauvoir, 1953, 15–16). For the oppressors, anyone who is "other" is not human, they are "things" (Freire, 1970, 57) to be conquered or consumed. This marginalization has a long history of being weaponized against women and people outside of the centers of societal power. Approximately 100,000 women healers were executed (Demos, 2008; in Ehrenreich & English, 2010, 14) during the "witch hunts" in Europe and North America. The fear and hatred of these women healers was misplaced, but it started the patriarchal removal of power from women in Euro-American society. In their place emerged the modern institution of medical science in the 19th century. This new institution of only men gained absolute political control of theory, practice, profits, and prestige. Men now controlled "who will live and who will die, who is fertile and who is sterile, who is 'mad' and who is sane" (Ehrenreich & English, 2010, 28). The institution was able to produce knowledge "from above"; placing scholars beyond the reach of the genuine world. Euro-American "science" focused upon elitist "peers" in the institution; effectively erasing the 3,000 years of clinical evidence, practical wisdom, and experience of women, Indigenous, Asian, and African traditional healers.

Please take a moment to slow down and reflect upon the list in this section again. Not just once, but five, ten, twenty more times. Feel how each element resonates within you, areas where you feel oppression, harm, or the need to hide your truth. Feel into the elements that you do not identify with, to practice being empathetic for the suffering that many people might experience overtly or silently. Consider the complexities of everyone's life. Remember that all people hold a concurrent mixture of joy and sorrow.

Even with "good" intentions; pause, reflect, and ask the person or group before assuming or taking action

The National Association of Social Workers (2021) and the American Psychological Association's feminist code evaluation (1999) brought attention to the discriminatory power differentials between people or groups. "The image of 'overlapping axes of oppression' (which is central to the metaphor of intersectionality) suggests an understanding of these processes of domination as detached from each other" (Erel, 2010, 73). This is incorrect, as the concurrent forms of interdependent discrimination are "experienced simultaneously" (Combahee River Collective, 1977, 213). The socio-economic stresses compound in an exponential manner, much worse than any individual or additive sum. Some discrete aspects of power differential discrimination that might be interdependent for clients are: age; experience, social standing, seniority, fame; class, money, poverty, and (un)employment; incarceration or (il)legality; religious (dis)belief, spirituality; political belief; national origin, nationality, citizenship, or immigration status; race, ethnicity, culture, heritage; assigned sex at birth; gender identity or expression; sexual orientation; single, (non)monogamous, or marital status; physical presence; skin tone, hair texture, visual aesthetic, fashionableness; bodily and cognitive ability; health or psychiatric diagnosis; and other forms of social injustice that are experienced as tensions in the mind, spirit, and body.

Some people have massive privilege, yet they also hold some amount of suffering. Some people that are massively discriminated against and oppressed still appreciate great joy in their life. Queen through street punk, kindergartener through president, physician through patient all exist upon a spectrum, a balance. No one has moral superiority over another. As stated above, not with wealth, education, chronology, nor any other element is anyone ever above another.

People being different from each other is what creates value. The homogenous "melting pot" legacy has caused harm for long enough. Striving for a statistical norm ignores the wonder of our differences. Utter equality would be mind-numbingly boring narcissistic nightmare. Relish the complexity and nuance that make all people unique. Differences allow ways for people to help each other learn, grow, and thrive. Some people would appreciate temporary scaffolding or long-term assistance to support their different needs. All people have the right to decline offers of assistance, whether other people assume to believe that they need help. Savior complex coupled with moral superiority can help people in ways that access was denied or perpetuate massive harm. Pause, reflect, and ask the person or group before assuming or taking action.

One of the main intents of sexual attitude restructuring or reassessment (SAR), a requirement of AASECT certification, is to get beyond the assumptions and privileges (McIntosh, 1988) that individuals might hold, and to understand that the lived experiences of different people are valid. These are opportunities for transformational thinking and being (Koltko-Rivera, 2004; Mezirow, 1997). SAR's transformational training is greatly important because many sexuality professionals are acculturalized in the moral taboos (Rubin, 1984) of society that prefer to keep the core topics of our work; sensuality and sexuality, sequestered to private enchanted mystery, instead of genuine visceral reality (Irvine, 2014; Plummer, 2012). Sexual care inhabiting the domains of desire, excitement, danger, dread and fear borders upon the erotic (Irvine, 2014; 2015; Twigg, 2011), which brings discomfort to many ill-trained professionals. Policy makers and academic training programs have been puritanically drawing the line of what is "allowable" (Rubin, 1984), which privileges and legitimizes some forms of knowledge, while marginalizing and erasing other lineages (Irvine, 2014).

The roots of "othering" knowledge and "appropriate" practice originated with the Victorian Era (1837–1901), and has been built upon ancient Greek foundations. Plato (c.330BCE) had prioritized the senses of sight and hearing for learning. He had denigrated taste, smell, and touch as being unworthy of intellectual consideration due to the potential of them bringing about pleasurable experiences (Moulton, 2010, 122), which he believed to be impediments for higher intellectual understanding. This privileging of vision has led to Hollywood and Madison Avenue's superficial objectification of sex (Fine & McClelland, 2006). Victorian ideals came up with a diabolical plan to limit women in the work place, similar to how medical institutions usurped the power of earth-based women healers. Moral connections were constructed between class, service, women, race, and sexuality to pollution and dirt (Attwood, 2007). The Victorians entitled the classist "Heart of Society" to remain pure, while assigning working-class women the undesirable "nether" regions that approach sin and temptation (Twigg, 2011). Professionals, who work with their intellect, were to be considered superior to the working-class that plunged their hands into the unclean scourge of society (Moutlton, 2010, 120). Most of the short-duration, part-time, low-paid, temporary, and peripheral laborers in the Victorian era were youth, women, and people of color (Barker & Jane, 2016, 168). Due to the intensity of their working hours and dismal living conditions, there were occasional "lapses in neatness, which were taken to be the equivalent of moral lapses" (Attwood, 2007). The evil twin of idealized femininity; "the succubus (whore, slut, concubine, witch) was the earthy, sensual, and frankly lusty woman who had traded respectability for sexual exuberance" (Perel, 2017, 46). The "phallusy" has never been able to integrate women's power, intelligence, and sexuality into their operative systems. Understanding that the deep roots of hierarchy, contorted social-sexual meaning, and division of labor based upon class, gender, race, and age will help clarify the magnitude of inertia and resistance to change in sexological professional policy (Twigg, 2011) will be considered below.

Intimate Care Services

Current policy determining practice is harming the sexual wellness of clients. Elitism, in the form of division of labor (intelligent vs. manual) and differentiation between holy and dirty, saturates every one of the professional codes of ethics in relation to dual relationships and touch. Discussions of transference and counter-transference often swirl around these topics. However, meta-cognition of societal stigma, bias, and foreclosed assignment of erotic meaning are not actively employed in the professional community. The nursing profession is very aware that personal care is integral to working successfully with clients. This arduous emotional labor was relegated to those of lower societal status (Twigg, 2011). To closely work physically and emotionally with a client requires a recognition of the personhood of the client, the visceral materiality of the suffering body. The work creates an energetic and practical intimacy; where one needs to effectively become entwined with the client. Yet, even though this emotional connection, sensitivity, and expression are inherent to quality work; that very same emotional intimacy is codified to be "unprofessional" (ibid.) and challenging of the prescriptive ways of acting in role theory.

The policy around this is based upon classism and pathologization. Most policies regulate dual relationships during current work, and some additionally delineate connections with close relations, partnerships, and sometimes friends based upon assumed risk of having diminished objectivity (AAMFT, 2015; AASECT, 2014; ACA, 2014; AMA, 2016; BACP, 2018; NASW, 2021). Multiple policies (AAMFT, 2015; AASECT, 2014; ACA, 2014; APA, 1999; BACP, 2018; NASW, 2021) also caution, limit, or preclude ever working with someone that the professional knew prior to potential care service provision. All of the mental health and some of the medical professions regulate relationships after the termination of services (AAMFT, 2015; AANP, 2015; AASECT, 2014; ACA, 2014; ACOG, 2018; AOA, 2022; APA, 1999; BACP, 2018; NASW, 2021; TCA, 2015). American Counseling Association (2014) requires a minimum five years of differentiation between professional work and potential future platonic or sexual relations, while the American Psychological Association (1999) stipulates two years, and the American Association of Naturopathic Physicians (2015) only one year. All recommend high caution, introspection, and potential supervisory review. The classist piece comes in when comparing how potential dual relationships are regulated with students and supervisees. Of the thirteen professional organizations, only five (AAMFT, 2015; AASECT, 2014; ACA, 2014; BACP, 2018; NASW, 2021) state that relations are not allowed while one has supervisory control over another. Only one precludes potential future relations (AASECT, 2014), and one disallows connection with their close relations or partnerships (AAMFT, 2015). Note that the American Nursing Association (2015) does not regulate the issue; even though they take great lengths to speak about protecting nurses due to a legacy of harm from sexual harassment, propositioned or actualized dual relationships amongst colleagues.

The great contrast in how clients are treated differently in these dual relationship policies, as opposed to students and supervisees, demand critique. Clients, students, and supervisees generally all pay for the professional services that they receive. Clients often have a longer duration of time and money investment that students or supervisees. This is potentially where the paradox comes into play. The classist elevation of the professional above client, and the a priori assumption and stigmatization of "brokenness" of the client in need of temporary or long-term care is the issue. The very core of why clients seek sex therapy or education is to address past trauma, grief tending, and mutually self-determined fulfilling relationships. Sexological professionals are expected to have been trained to successfully assist clients in these pursuits (Schiller, 1973; Binik & Meana, 2009). Should it not also be required that professionals have integrated their training personally, and therefore have the practical wisdom in their own personal actions? Even though "intimacy skills (e.g., social, emotional, sexual), intimate relationships, interpersonal relationships and family dynamics" and "pleasure enhancement skills" (AASECT 2022.csc; 2022.cse; 2022.cst) are required, there is no expectation, and certainly no vetting, that sexological professionals have integrated these skills for practical use in their own relationships. Institutional compartmentalization of mind from body often causes sensuality and scholarship to become mutually exclusive (Nelson, 2017, 231). Nzegwu pokes fun at the fallacy of professionals by sharing the story of a person being perplexed by "how anyone with so much book knowledge and a 'doctor' title could be so inept" sexually (2011, 265). Sándor Ferenczi states that in psycho-sexual work; "our patients gradually become better analyzed [and educated] than we ourselves" (1949, 198). Following this thought, it would be logical to deduce that the "problem" with dual relationships is not the risk of exploitation, coercion, harming, and/or influencing a client away from self-determination. The problem is the ineptitude of professional training, or the requirement of enough duration in the training process to allow for integration of intellectualism into embodied actions. This is why sexological professionals need to have further training around touch and the compassionate care inherent in genuine interpersonal relationships (discussed further below). Academic programs churn out professionals with "book smarts," but not meta-cognition, compassion, nor compersion.

The stigma of compassionate connection is heightened in the erotic borderlands of touch. Even more terrifying than the taboos of sexual identities and orientations is the potential of crossing the erotic line into or beyond the "erotic DMZ [demilitarized zone], the barrier against scary sex will crumble and something unspeakable will skitter across" (Rubin, 1984, 282). Even the slightest whiff of sexuality, and our primitive brains devolve to a place of fear, that our "wild nature" will be uncontrollable (Nelson, 2017, 235). Touch-deprived acculturalization, institutionalized training, and dysregulation converge to codify touch as sinfully erotic, even when it can be quite the opposite in reality (Tune, 2001). Instead of allowing for the potential of loving care and beneficence, policies assume harm will be perpetrated due to the field of sexuality's association with the "Dark Triad" of Machiavellianism (cynical manipulation), psychopathy (non-empathetic thrill-seeking), and narcissism (grandiose entitlement) (Bolelli, 2019; Paulhus & Williams, 2002; Kaufman, 2019). People intuitively know from birth that touch can be healthy. Therefore, many practitioners are actually touching their clients, however it is done clandestinely (Tune, 2001; Owen & Gillentine, 2011; Harrison, 2012) and without the professional training of the skilled paraprofessionals described below.

Ethic Codes for Sensuality Para-Professionals

Acknowledging that holistic care requires connection and positive touch, the following section looks at 12 policies of sensuality para-professions that integrate these into their professional services in a range of methods. The American Massage Therapy Association (AMTA, 2010), American Physical

Therapy Association (APTA, 2010), and National Certification Board for Therapeutic Massage & Bodywork (NCBTMB, 2017) all employ touch at the core of their work that is specifically non-erotic and non-relational. The Kink Education Code of Conduct Collective (KECC, 2019) recognizes that touch and relationships are part of genuine life and education, while developing strong practices around communication, consent, and role-modeling. The Association of Certified Sexological Bodyworkers (ACSB, 2014) and Certified Cuddlers (CC, 2016) recognize the importance of genuine erotic and connective experiences, while maintaining boundaries, one-sidedness to the interactions, and general avoidance of erogenous zones. The International Professional Surrogates Association (IPSA, 2020) and Surrogate Partner Collective (SPC, 2022) also holds strong boundaries, while allowing for more transparency around eroticism, full-body integration, and actions that are potentially therapeutic.

Three of the organizations firmly stipulate against relationships (AMTA, 2010; APTA, 2010; NCBTMB, 2017). This is in part to politically differentiate between "professional" massage and erotic "full-service" massage that is possible with some sex workers. ACSB, CC, and KECC all caution about the potential for exploitation, coercion, or harming a client; yet recognize that positive mindful relationships are possible. The CC stipulates that if one is sexual (versus the sensuality intrinsic to cuddling) with a client, that the client cannot be a client again for 90 days. No other organization in this section has preclusions about prior relationships. The NCBTMB allows for post-professional relationships after a six-month hiatus. Only the IPSA and SPC have strong opposition to post-professional relationships, specifically because navigating the completion of an intimate sexual relationship is core to the potential services that are offered in client care. None of these organizations stipulate about dual relationships with the friends, relations, or partners of clients. Due to the marginalization of sex work, there is no quasi-legalization of ethics at this time. However, the Sex Workers' Rights Advocacy Network (SWAN, 2021) forecasts how such policies might develop when the work is decriminalized in the future.

For the purposes of this discussion, it seems important to differentiate between the BodyWork that might be provided by an acupuncturist, beauty worker, erotic telephone worker, esthetician, hair stylist, massage therapist, physiotherapist, reflexologist, shamanic healer, somatic bodyworker, tattoo artist, or yoga teacher; versus embodied work provided by an escort, film actor, professional dominant, prostitute, stripper, surrogate, tantrika, and webcam performer. BodyWork focuses labor explicitly upon the bodies of clients for an exchange of mutual value. The labor provided in BodyWork is not purposefully erotic, although it can spur erotic fantasy for the client. While Plummer (1975) might muse that hair styling can be a sexually erotic act, for the purposes of discussion this chapter will differentiate between the services sold and the unintended potentiality of the experience for inherently erotic bodies. Sexual service providers enable consensual exchange of core emotions, connections, relationships, or performances that are hegemonically defined to be part of private, personal, or family relationships; such as caring, friendship, and sensuality as a potentially economic sustainable activity (MacFarlane, 2017; SWAN, 2021, 14). Some providers identify as Sex Workers. There is a range in the legality of these services across the globe.

> Although some people have criticized the practice [of surrogate partner work] as being only a thinly veiled form of prostitution, others see it as an important means of helping people who are unable to find a partner who will accompany them in sex therapy.
>
> (Masters & Johnson, 1982, 499)

Many people in society might exchange gifts, currency, or support for implicit sexual favors and not consider themselves to be sex workers; such as trophy wives or hegemonic dating (Harcourt & Donovan, 2005; Stanger, 2017), that might trade sexuality for food, shelter, or other needs. In all of these forms of relationship exchange, boundaries might need to be firmly held if a client holds a false privileged assumption that the client has a right to access or express their non-mutual erotic expectations upon the worker. Worker risk can range from street harassment, to sexual harassment or criminal assault. All workers need a living wage, consensual selection of clients for differential services provided, and access to health- and community-based services (Harcourt & Donovan, 2005). Understanding the difference between explicit consent and implicit assumptions will help the reader understand the further discussion about professional ethics below.

Multicultural Sexuality Healthcare Practices

Beauchamp and Childress (2019, 2) start their lengthy 512-page investigation of biomedical ethics by extolling ten virtues: nonmalevolence, honesty, integrity, conscientiousness, trustworthiness, fidelity, gratitude, truthfulness, lovingness, and kindness. Most of these virtues are examined in great depth, except for the omission of lovingness and kindness. Love is briefly mentioned twice in the tome, as the "ethics of care emphasizes traits valued in intimate personal relationships such as sympathy, compassion, fidelity, and love. Caring refers to care for, emotional commitment to, and willingness to act on behalf of persons with whom one has a significant relationship" (ibid., 30). Not emphasizing the importance of love, care, and kindness might satisfy nonmaleficence's complacency. However, professionals can strive toward the proactive nature of beneficence. A reason that love has not been discussed further is because the relationship being loving or caring is presumed irrelative to morality (ibid., 62). It is quite likely that Beauchamp and Childress did not want to take the professional risk of appearing ridiculous, ascientific, or even anti-scientific in proposing the importance of love

(Freire, 1970, 26). Similar to sex, the consumerist marketing of love as something that all people must possess is everywhere in popular media, art, and literature as a deceitful illusion, pastiche, or simulacra. It is one of the highest cultural goals, yet often left in a state of mystery. This has not always been the case in the United States, and certainly not across the globe.

The roots of sexual shame and stigma reach back to the Roman conquest (c.275) of all lands adjacent to the Mediterranean Sea. Being an ascetic Christian, Saint Augustine believed there was innate evil in sexual desire and bound to the material world. "His legacy of shame, fear of the body, and suspicion of its desires is with us today" (Schermer Seller, 2017, 33), and potentially influences all of the cultures descendent of the Roman Empire's post-Augustine colonization of Europe, the Middle East, and Africa (Wiseman, 2008). This was reinforced by Pope Benedict XV in 1918 with the Pio-Benedictine Code (aka "Canon Law") to define what was sexually "allowable," thereby only "legitimizing" pro-creative sexual acts (Stayton, 1992, 204). The religious stigmatization of sexuality has created much confusion.

> Contrary to the belief of many Christians, the writers of the Bible were not as concerned about the acts of sexual intercourse as they were about human relationships and the motives and consequences of sexual acts… Nowhere does [Jesus], even in his teaching of self-denial, condemn sexual pleasure. His concern is always the wholeness, the spiritual well-being, and the loving relationships of people.
>
> (Stayton, 2002)

To further contextualize what Anglo-Saxons privileged to teach in medical schools and codify in biomedical ethics during the formation of the AMA (1847), APA (1892), ANA (1896), and AOA (1897), sexuality professionals need to culturally recognize the homogenizing zeitgeist of nearly 12 million people immigrating to a country in political turmoil. America and Mexico were at war until 1848, and the conflicts over slavery and land had eventually led to the Civil War (1861–1865). The federal government enacted the Reservation Policy of 1851, forcing Indigenous people to limited locations, unceding ancestral and spiritual connection to land and seasonal migration. Many wars have followed, such as the Sioux Wars (1854–1876). The criminal treatment of Indigenous people became politically known as the "Century of Dishonor" (Jackson, 1881); which had caused the government to retaliate with the Dawes Act (1887) that fractured tribes and destroyed Indigenous culture. Chinese, Black, and Mexican labor built the transcontinental railroad (1862–1869). The Emancipation Proclamation officially ended slavery in 1863, while the transatlantic slave trade continued until 1866. Howard University became the first school to have a medical program for Black students in 1868. In 1882, to free up jobs for Anglo-Saxons, the federal Chinese Exclusion Act stopped the immigration of Chinese people for nearly a century. It was not until 1981 that the American College of Traditional Chinese

Medicine had started to teach one of the first non–Anglo-Saxon approaches with five element medicine. The formation of the American Association of Naturopathic Physicians followed four years later. The American Traditional Chinese Medicine Association (ATCMA) was recently registered in 2016.

There are many relationships between contemporary feminism, midwifery, and multicultural sensuality. Nzegwu (2011) explains that the domination of men in Euro-American eroticism centers the preference for linguistic, theoretical, and contrived perspectives of eros. She expands upon Diop's research that as civilizations spread from the fertile crescent there was a split in sensual-spiritual ways of being. As people migrated, the nomadic ways of life that led to the Indo-European society created a sense of insecurity and practices of subjugation. Conversely, those who had remained, and slowly developed in the southern cradle of Africa, had maintained a connection with nature that inspired a peaceful and connective sense of sexual-spirituality. Òsunality creates connections with all of life, creation, and transformation that includes Indo-European conceptualizations of "sexuality," and much more. This sense of connection inspires the virtue of ubuntu (humaneness), which embraces and connects all diverse beings in a universal bond (Ramose, 1999; in Tamale, 2011).

Interestingly, the Indigenous cultures of what is now called North America embrace a similar connective sensual-spirituality to Òsunality while embracing migratory culture. This supports Nzegwu's sensual futurism, yet questions some of Diop's research in relation to attachment theory and migration. Nelson (2017, 235–238) describes the Indigenous closeness to non-humanism, where animals, plants, cloud beings, the wind, stars, and what are mistaken in Anglo-Saxon eyes as inanimate sticks and rocks are sexual beings to share in mutually beneficial carnal relations. The panopticon of modern psychiatry (Foucault, 1978) discount these holistic pansexual visceral connections to the more-than-human world as insanity (Roszak, 1996, 22; in Nelson, 2017). An important Indigenous virtue is to question the illusion of the psycho-sexual panopticon and seek one's own truth (Houser, 2006, 52). The Mi'kmaq seek to embody kesalttimkewey (deep love) and kesalk (spirit of love) as a gravitational life force to bind all people in kinship (Henderson, 2015; in Nelson, 2017, 248–249). The native people of Hawai'i vibrantly embrace akahai (kind tenderness), lokahi (harmonic unity), o'lu'olu (agreeable pleasantness), ha'aha'a (modest humility), and ahonui (persevering patience) in life (Le & Jackman, 2022, 5).

The Shinto beliefs of South-East Asia similarly aspired for a sensual-spirituality with nature. Kami, spiritual essence, strives to unite the conscious sense of self with the environment, thereby freeing the unconscious to flow freely (Kasai, 2009). The Buddhist way of dissolving worldly understanding to a state of enlightenment is closer to Shinto than the body-hating precepts of Saint Augustine's ascetic Christianity. Being present in solo or partnered sensuality is divine, and a glimpse if not a path to enlightenment. From these sprang forth Confucianism and Hinduism. In Ferrer's study of compersion, sympathetic joy for other beings (2021, 80), he speaks of the four brahmavihara values of mudita (joy), metta (loving kindness), karuna (compassion), and upeksha (equanimity). In this Hindi way of being, the individual is both centered and dematerialized. The Anglo-Saxon "ego self" is impermanent, and by each individual striving toward enlighten-ment, the collective will blossom (Houser, 2006, 68). Similar to African ubuntu, as Shinto and Buddhism had transformed into Confucianism, a core value of inclusion pervaded society. This does not negate the self-determinism aspects of Anglo-Saxon precepts of autonomy, but does prefer collective connection over individualism. The desire for inclusion strives for connective dual-relationships. Circa 770BCE (hundreds of years prior to Aristotle and Plato in Greece), folk traditions of witchcraft transformed from sorcery to prognosis and experience-based knowledge, with profes-sional skills and ethics being taught in medical schools (Zhang & Cheng, 2000). However, Chinese medicine continued to focus upon the "moral commitment to love people and free them from suffering through personal caring and medical treatment" (ibid.). Clients are to be treated as lovingly as family, knowing that connection and love strengthens one's desire to provide care wisely. For over 2500 years, Confucianism informed the moral ideology of Chinese practitioners of the healing arts (Tsai, 1999). Tz'u (compassion), jen (humaneness), ren (love), and li (closeness) com-posed a harmonious beneficence. During the Qing dynasty (1644–1912), Neo-Confucianism had revived some earlier Buddhist and Taoist ways. However, with the Xinhai Revolution (1911), the Republic of China was founded and soon had embraced bio-science principles similar to Anglo-Saxons (Chiang, 2018).

Coming full-circle, contemporary feminist psychology focuses upon compassionate personal care of clients, which assumes creating genuine and emotional connections; instead of the abstract generalized justice systems of "reason" and "right" actions (Houser, 2006, 41). Care is a fluid and ever-changing continuum of internal and external worlds seeking balance (APA, 1999). The care provider is to be actively involved in community to create a sense of equality and empowerment for clients. Consciousness Raising (CR) groups were formed to support care provider's personal needs and develop-ment. As the women in these groups shared their personal and professional life experiences, a sense of solidarity emerged. An understanding that the world cannot change, and the trauma experienced by individuals or col-lectively cannot heal if people struggle alone. The path to change is through connection and collaboration.

Coalition Building

A love revolution blossomed with the visionary leadership of Lorde (1979), Dodson (1974), McIlvenna (1975), the Combahee River Collective (1977), and many more. The voices and experiences of the marginalized "others" became re-centered and prioritized as sources of trusted wisdom for sexual healthcare service (APA, 2018, 4). This is the revolution of women, Indigenous, Black, North African, Latinx, Asian, Middle Eastern, Turkish, lesbian, gay, pansexual, trans*, queer, intersex, asexual, celibate, two-spirit, kinky, spectrums of cognitive and physical abilities, immigrants, refugees, and people across all ages, regardless of wealth or historical power. The safety of identity affinity will help along the incremental pathway to equitable liberation. However, this is a revolution to include everyone, as multiculturally discussed above, or the harm of oppressors will be perpetrated by exclusion and discrimination. This is a revolution prioritizing love instead of resistance (Tario, 2019). Freire (1970, 50; 1978, 8) beckons the oppressor to be part of these solidary actions; as active inclusion will shift the abstraction of the "other" to embrace the humaneness of tangible persons that have been deprived of voice, cheated, and unjustly treated.

As individuals coalesce into a revolutionary "salad bowl" of "us" the many voices will need to negotiate boundaries and agreements. A neo-"We" will show-up with a plethora of moralistic agendas. "We" will hopefully find common ground to scribe neo-ethical ways of living together in society. However, Rich (1971) and Lorde (1979) have cautioned "us" not to repeat oppression under the guise of false liberation. Euro-American sexuality professionals have all been saturated in the Roman and Anglo-Saxon sexual colonizing language. For many, all that is known is this oppressor's language, and yet to work together, this is the language that "we" know to start with. If the neo-"We" perpetuates the old ways of being, people might temporarily be able to "beat" the oppressors at their own game, but it will not bring about genuine change. People self-oppress because they have been psychosexually colonized by oppressive "morality" (APA, 2018, 8). Sexuality professionals can throw away some of the oppressing "Master's" harmful tools such as "objective distancing," to instead embrace connection. Yet, people can also embrace the importance of Anglo-Saxon self-determination and beneficence. Sexuality professionals can venture toward more-than-humanism, by embracing the roots of ubuntu, jen, upeksha, tz'u, karuna, mudita, li, lokahi, ren, metta, akahai, kesalttimkewey, kesalk, o'lu'olu, ha'aha'a, ahonui, care, and inclusivity. This is a process of lateral and transformational thinking (Mezirow, 1997; hooks, 1984). Lateral thinking is approaching a circumstance with one's existing tools in a fresh way. Such as turning a pair of pliers on the side to use it as a hammer. Transformational thinking is the chrysalis process, where the spirit of being continues (such as humaneness) without the detritus husk of what needs to be shed (humanism) to embody a new self. Pre-colonial (c.1778) Hawaiian society embraced mo'okū'auhau, a fluid and inclusive sense of "We," which continues in the present day recognizing genuine "power" roots in connecting our individual story, worldview, and values with all "family" that shares land (Le & Jackman, 2022, 5). The state of Hawai'i (1996) embracing the Spirit of Aloha in legislature, provides great hope for the future of biomedical ethics.

Okun (1999) highlights the aspects of kyriarchy that are deeply ingrained and need excision: perfectionism, urgency, defensiveness, consumerism, codification, rightness, superiority, binaries, power, fear of vulnerability, individualism, objectivity, and comfort. Each one of these are enticing and can draw one away from the discomfort of metamorphic transformation. However, if all people seek to jettison the oppressive familiar ways, the incremental process of unlearning will be deeply uncomfortable and difficult (Tamale, 2011, 5). Many people will cling to the comfortable latticework of what has been known (Takacs, 2003). The often quoted "Medice, cura te ipsum," physician, heal thyself (Jesus; in Luke, 85, 4.23) was a passage about being in the frightening wilderness of temptatious "sin", to learn from the unknown, emerge with new found wisdom, and to bring love, touch, and connection to heal everyone (ibid., 4.40). However, this is not an easy task, as much fear of the "wild" continues to this day. Society teaches people to keep on their medieval armor, to be perfect, strong, independent, and never vulnerable.

Love and Vulnerability

Of the neo–retro-values (care, closeness, compassion, equanimity, humane-ness, inclusivity, joy, and love), it is love that potentially needs the most affirmative action. Beauchamp and Childress (2019, 2) had recognized the central importance of love as an Anglo-Saxon virtue. Bioscience is not just about saving lives, it is a moral commitment to love our clients (Zhang & Cheng, 2000). The panopticon of self-oppression will gaslight people into thinking that love is a "crazy" value to practice professionally (Foucault, 1978; Rorty, 1991). Harlow (1958) mocks modern psycho-sexologists by noting that professional repression of love as a virtue stands in sharp con-trast with the common understanding of many famous and "normal" peo-ple. This is mostly due to professional confusion upon the meaning that has been placed upon the act of loving. Lee (1977) defines love in sex categories: eros (physical), ludus (playfulness), storge (companionship), mania (obses-sive), agape (altruistic), and pragma (statistically beneficial). The version of love that is commercialized, and permeates professional understanding of love's potential, is eros. While eros is defined by Lee to focus upon the pursuit of an aesthetic archetype, the visual longing is intertwined with lust-ful visceral physicality. This confusion around eros is what will be discussed below in bell hooks' classroom experience. The forms of love that sexual-ity professionals need to develop fluency with are agape and storge. Storge is a "slowly developing affection and companionship" (ibid.) that comes with mutually practicing vulnerability, dissolving of ego, and building trust. Agape is a form of altruism where one gently cares for another from a place of core value, and not with expectation of reciprocity. Harlow (1958) encourages the investigation of love, regardless of its potential "improper" intimate and personal nature, as a wondrous, deep, tender, and rewarding state. Capitalism has distorted the genuine nature of love (Freire, 1970, 89). Love is an act of courage. Love is taking risks in the face of potential criticism and fear. Love is being vulnerable.

> I understand my most important role as a practitioner is to love and be love. Love in this sense is an act and attitude of body, mind, spirit, and emotions... I love the receivers' spirits, with an unconditional love that could be called agape. I stand in spirit and greet their spirits in a state of wonder and amazement. I am agape, wide open, as I experience the joy of working with erotic energy.
>
> (Jesse, 2020, 35)

The need for a spectrum of love and touch burns within all people. If only appeased via marketing, social media, and superficiality, that fire can become a destructive force. The pent-up energy venting in forms of non-consent, abuse, assault, and even self-harm. However, if the metabolic fire is appeased incrementally with an assortment of love and touch, the spirit will thrive creatively.

There is an additional Anglo-Saxon worry that objectivity will be compromised if a prior or concurrent caring relationship occurs with a client, friend, family, or partner. Okun (1999) challenges the objective vs. emotional binary, and states that the very notion of neutrality is a delusion. Emotions are not inherently destructive nor irrational, and the assumption privileges linear "logical" thinking. Freire (1970, 64), hooks (1984, 21), Swan (2002), and Brown (2013) all agree that empowerment cannot occur if those holding power are not vulnerable. The sharing of vulnerability allows the client, student, supervisee, or friend to recognize and compassionately engage the professional's imperfect humanity. It also directly addresses the power imbalance between the professional and the client's capacity for agentic self-determination. Ferenczi (1949, 200) proposes that by admitting imperfection, sharing mistakes, honestly endeavoring to not repeat harm in the future, and discussing pathways explored for healing any harm done, will help a client feel confidence in the professional's integrated skills. "It is this confidence that establishes the contrast between the present and the unbearable traumatogenic past, the contrast which is absolutely necessary for the patient in order to enable him to re-experience the past no longer as hallucinatory reproduction" (ibid.). Trust comes from sharing potential risk without harm having been experienced. Vulnerability is a form of selfless love that can allow the client to feel a range of compassion and compersion for each other's humanity and personal growth. Swan (2002) recommends to establish a baseline of comfort and connection with clients, which will help create trust for the professional's veracity and fidelity. Then be open to questions from the client, while holding unblurring autonomous boundaries. While "No means No" for the general population, professionals implicitly agree to a burden of less privacy (KECC, 2019, 23), and unpacking the "No" in order to teach the client is required.

Any blurred area can be clarified with the declaration of a boundary, at least a simple explanation of why the boundary is required, and affirmation of any boundary or vulnerability that the client reciprocally shares.

Marginalization

As sexological professionals it is important to frame the dual relationship dialogue with an understanding of discrimination. The privileged assumption of the "zero dual relationships" policy is that there are a plethora of social and support options. This is not the case if one has been marginalized. The policy assumes that if a client is going to the same venue, that the professional can go to a different and equal one. This assumption works if the professional and client are both white, cis-heterosexual, monogamous, Christian, vanilla, wealthy, urban, and without any mobility or sensory restrictions. If the client or professional have intersectional marginalizations, the options can shrink exponentially, and the Venn diagram of options for the two individuals can quickly overlap. It is also important to note that clients might seek an affinity professional with similar marginalizations or community networks. The number of social or recreational options for marginalized populations at this time, in even the largest of international cities, is limited. Therefore, it is almost guaranteed that clients will bump into the professional at a support group, bath house, munch, or play party. "Normalizing" the belief that witnessing each other in these situations is harmful ignores this reality for marginalized people, and perpetuates the stigmatization of those being marginalized. It assumes that sexuality is shameful, and seeing someone in a potentially sexually charged environment is near criminal. Key to humaneness is that many people buy groceries, socialize, giggle, fuck, and do things awkwardly sometimes. Cherishing and centering how people live in all of the visceral complexity of our bodies challenges the very constructs of how power was stolen from the marginalized (hooks, 1984, 137). Clients learn from professional's personal lives as well as from what they experience in the clinical setting (KECC, 2019, 6). Witnessing how a client interacts with other people platonically through to erotically allows professionals to understand the nuance of where further education and practice might best serve the client in their chosen lifestyle. The power structures, particularly in academia and professional organizations, continue to privilege those who can deny the nature of their bodies and sexuality. The ACA (2014), ANA (2015), and NASW (2021) policies do an excellent job of engaging the topic of social justice, and how this needs to change. Integration of how intersectional marginalization affects professionals and clients on a personal level is highly advised. Particularly upon how autonomous decision making is affected by diminished capacity and/or agency. Plus, an understanding of how one's access to touch and caring interpersonal individual and communal interactions is affected by intersectional social marginalization.

Touch

With touch being central to professional practice, and recognizing that there are greatly different affects from positive, neutral, or negative types of touch, it is essential that the mechanisms are understood (Estabrooks & Morse, 1992). Many evidence-based researchers have clearly shown that the benefits of positive touch greatly outweigh the risks that cause some professional anxiety (Harrison, 2012; Owen & Gillentine, 2011). Touch is a multi-dimensional experience that involves the voice of the toucher, the way that the toucher positions their body in space, posture, the intention of the toucher, and the affect experienced by the touchee (Estabrooks & Morse, 1992). The effect experienced by the touchee can match the intention of the toucher, or it can vary greatly due to temporal, societal, and personal context. However, touch is essential, more than any other of the physical senses and experiences (Moulton, 2010, 125). Therefore, the author would recommend that all sexuality professionals engage basic touch training, with the option of advanced explorations. Without the primal nature of touch, the species would literally no longer exist. More importantly, touch can be an act of love and care (Kennedy & Dean, 1995, 19; Jesus; in Luke, 85, 4.23) that transcends words and other more overt actions. Touch conveys positive care or cold neutrality more effectively than any verbal method. The effects of touch are at the very core of Sexuality Healthcare Services.

Czimbal and Zadikov (1991), Estabrooks and Morse (1992), Jesse (2020), Kosierb and Bilodeau (2020), Routasalo (1999), Willison and Masson (1986), and others have found multiple benefits to utilizing touch therapeutically. Even more effective than the "Permission (P)" aspect of the Annon (1976) P.LI.SS.IT. model, touch compliments verbal communication by creating a form of recognized acceptance and solidarity that helps heal lowered self-esteem due to otherness, erasure, and marginalization. Not all people have access to consensual touch for free, and it is a compassionate service to provide clients (Stanger, 2017). Positive professional touch experiences can increase trust and openness. Similar to how Ferenczi (1949, 200) proposes to heal the "traumatogenic past" in connective relationships, touch conveys a sense of caring, closeness, and strengthens bonds. "Touch is far more than a cutaneous sensation; it opens the way for a trustful, respectful co-existence between therapist and patient, and in tandem with movement enters a dance-like progress in whose silent, leisured pace there are healing possibilities" (Bjorbækmo, 2016, 10). Touch is a "ground control" to calm a client, transition from being stuck in their head or drifting in fantasy to present-moment bodily awareness, which can allow unrecognized emotions held in the body to emerge. Kosierb and Bilodeau (2020) and Willison and Masson (1986) have found positive professional touch to be effective in treating clients suffering from grief, neglect, depression, trauma, acute distress, physical and emotional abuse. "Professionals can enhance the quality of the service they provide by understanding the therapeutic value of touch" (Czimbal & Zadikov, 1991, 101). Understanding these professional skills, receiving training, practicing, and asking what, if any, type of touch a client desires, will greatly advance our profession.

Culture of Fear

Touch has been firmly lodged in the societal contempt and fear of "getting dirty" as it is inherently visceral, and teeters upon empathic kinship (Nelson, 2017, 232; Attwood, 2007). Organizational policies generally infantilize the consent capacity of clients. The policies consider clients and research subjects informed consent, and those of close relatives, guardians, or significant others, to be moot. Most policies eradicate all forms of touch, out of fear that a few sexualized forms of touch such as kissing, penetration, and pelvic/chest genital area contact might transpire. The societal sexual imperative that desire or acknowledgment of eros must lead to coercive, harmful, and abusive sexual actions is harm in itself. Not all behaviors are sexual (Plummer, 1975) nor should be sexualized (Gagnon & Simon, 1973). Professional training should allow any sexual or sexualized affects to be addressed in a way that would promote trust and "traumatogenic" healing. Fear and risk avoidance has undermined the ability to facilitate sexual wellness. The Anglo-Saxon bias of professional asceticism is defining the "sinfulness" of the intervention, not the actual touch affects (Tune, 2001, 168; Drescher, 2013). Sexuality professionals need to transcend the recursive hegemonic monologue (Kennedy & Dean, 1995, 20–21) that biases our ability and comfort to touch and be touched. Professionals and the lay public can work together to proactively satiate societal touch starvation.

Clients and professionals who have been raised with warm and loving touch tend to be comfortable with touch and incorporate it unconsciously into behaviors across the spectrum of their lives (Estabrooks & Morse, 1992). Some professionals raised with touch, confront internal conflict when told by professional groups that touch is not allowed. Others that have not been raised with touch can feel an uneasiness, which can be countered through somatic therapy and personal practice. There can even be unease due to the counter-transferred desire around potential touch, even if it is not actually an option. bell hooks has discussed her personal experience of assuming eroticism while teaching critical pedagogy to transgress assumptions about gender and sexuality (1984, 192–195). While in her professional space she found herself erotically drawn to a student, she was not academically prepared to handle the feelings that had stirred within her. She found herself in a paradox, in that professionals have the post-colonial expectation to "bring quality care and even 'love'" to students, but she was not prepared for the emergence of genuine eros in the professional space. What she had deduced is that the abundance and infinite possibilities of eroticism is limited when eros is assumed to only have hegemonic sexual meaning. This tunnel vision upon procreation, romanticism, and genital pleasure betrays our disconnection from more-than-humanism, to Òsun, Kami, and Kesalk, to animals, plants, and the nature that people are part. Please remember this when bringing touch into professional practice. Touch does not have implicit meaning. People propose meaning with the intention of their touch. People interpret meaning when receiving touch. Professionals can help clients navigate meaning making.

Somatic exercises allow the client to practice in the shallow end before taking the plunge into deeper waters with consensual adult relationships, since a "person learns to swim in the water, not in a library" (Freire, 1970, 137). In sensate focus and other touch exercises, clients recognize sensations and interpreted meanings, such as anxiety or arousal, as if they are inconsequential passing clouds in the open sky (Masters & Johnson, 1982, 488–489; Zal, 2022). Bring eros, love, and care into our work to authentically share intimacy with clients in the embodied practice exercises (ACSB, 2014, 5). However, this is mostly meant to be a unidirectional form of touching. The professional is the conduit of the intention, but not the consumer. Whether surrogate, bodyworker, therapist, or educator, any practice exercise is not meant to fulfill the desire for sexual connection (ibid.). If either the professional or client become physically aroused with perspiration, pelvic or chest tumescence, or anxiety, simply acknowledge the reaction and allow it to dissipate (CC, 2016), grow, or shift. There is zero goal or expectation. There is no "right" or "wrong" in the explorations. It is natural to feel something when touching another person. Newton's third law of dynamics states that energy from one body will radiate similarly in the body touched (1687; in Routasalo, 1999). Routasalo notes that the very nature of therapeutic touch is a mode of healing by influencing the client's energy fields. Willison and Masson advise that patterns of emotional or physical reaction can cause client transference desires or expectations with the professional. If one is clear about the intentions of the practice exercises, and one recognizes any feelings that emerge within oneself without feelings of counter-transference, then the "advantages of touch greatly outweigh the disadvantages in working through these intense reactions" (1986). Willison and Masson humorously convey that; "touch a paranoid and risk losing a tooth; touch a seductress and risk losing your license; touch a violent patient with a short fuse and risk losing everything" (Older, 1982, 201; in ibid.). This is why behavioral vetting of clients by a trained professional is central to the triadic care model. It is important to gauge a client's self-awareness of their sensual needs and desires; if the client is able to communicate with a level of clarity; is prone to harmful transference; and can respect the boundaries of others. Research has shown that "clients who were assertive enough to request touch were likely to have this need met outside therapy and consequently, touch was deemed less of a necessity" (Harrison, 2012). If a professional refers a client prematurely, this can be harmful to both the client and the receiving professional referee. Clients with less skills in these areas might also have less access to touch due to marginalization.

Trauma and shame freeze our bodies and disempower our voices. If clients can learn to speak their truth and ask for what they want in sexual situations, they will expand their capacity for pleasure. I encourage clients to intuit their boundaries and practice defending them. We explore how they can embody a sense of "Yes", "No", "Maybe", and "I changed my mind". We might work for many hours with the question, "How would you like to be touched?" Sinking into that question and feeling the answer from the inside can be a powerful learning experience, a way of exploring and developing an expanded container of consent that increases the possibilities of pleasure. With patient practice, clients learn to put an end to enduring, and to feel and speak their truth in erotic exchanges.

(Jesse, 2020, 23)

Triadic Collaboration

In a Triadic Model the collaborating trio of client and two differing professionals work together on a treatment plan to meet the care goals of the client. The professional collaborator assists a client learn and practice "social, emotional, and physical intimacy skills within a real-life environment" (SPC, 2022.el). Both professionals support the client's care goals in parallel and distinct ways. These services often benefit a client that feels an intimate relationship is inaccessible due to social anxiety, trauma, abuse, physical or cognitive differences (Stanger, 2017). Surrogacy has been limited to be temporary, clients must be "actively and concurrently engaged with a qualified collaborating clinician" (SPC, 2022.sc), and the professional work with the clinician precedes and extends beyond the time working with the surrogate (SPC, 2022.el). Some clients have access to general forms of touch or intimacy, and are wanting additional marginalized variations that are possible with a Professional Dominant. Some simply want to "out-source" touch as distinct from their primary intimate relationship (Kirschner, 2005). Working triadically has the potential of providing a client with a full range of services that meet their personal care goals, while respecting the differing training, practiced skill sets, and organizational boundaries of each professional. These professional collaborations also have the potential to legitimize the importance of the work. Kamala Harris (Vice-President of the United States at the time of this writing, and former Senator and California Attorney-General) stated; "If it's between consensual adults and referred by licensed therapists and doesn't involve minors, then it's not illegal" (1997). Harris' statement has added additional privilege to therapists' power over clients and other sexuality professionals in defining the scope of morality, taboos, and professionalism for client access to love, care, and touch. The Surrogate Partner Collective (2022.el) feels distinctly confident that therapists collaborating with surrogates will not place their licensure in jeopardy. "Although some people have criticized this practice [of surrogate partner work] as being only a thinly veiled form of prostitution, others see it as an important means of helping people" (Masters & Johnson, 1982, 499). With other stigmatized sex work professionals, the risks in providing client care are less clear in differing jurisdictions. This is why surrogacy has purposely, and ironically, removed the word "sex" from their nomenclature. Other forms of professional services do not have such regulation. Whether therapist, educator, counselor, surrogate, stripper, or ProDomme it is certainly not all about sex. It is about building a "foundation of self-awareness, healthy boundaries, good communication, relaxation, and positive body image" (SPC, 2022.el), along with a plethora of other valuable life skills. It is in the interest of professionals in areas of marginalized work to create sustainable triadic coalitions.

Consent

If touch is going to be part of the therapeutic process, the client and professional will need to understand, fully integrate, navigate, and practice consent. Policies often state that any touch must be client initiated. However, this assumes clients have the privileged full capacity and agency to initiate touch. Consent must allow for mutual self-determination of boundaries based upon clear understanding of the intent, type of touch, duration, location, intensity, frequency, and sensation potentiality (Zal, 2019; Routasalo, 1999). If there are power differentials or circumstances that can diminish the client's capacity or agency, the exercises should be postponed or terminated. Czimbal and Zadikov (1991, 39) offer the I.N.T.I.M.A.C.Y. mnemonics to determine if and how touch will be engaged: Intensity (emotional charge), Number (amount of touch), Time (length of touch), Intention (purpose of the touch), Mutual (common level of respect), Affection (tender feelings), Contact (kind of touch), and Yes! (explicit desire for touch). One of the authors of the KECC (2019) recommends to only negotiate by inclusion (Tiziano, 2021). Opt-in negotiation differs from opt-out processes, in that both people explicitly state what is allowable for the touch exercise. Anything not explicitly included and agreed upon is off limits; and not to be questioned, influenced, nor coerced further down the road. Both the professional and the client must agree that they are not playing a game of challenging boundaries (CC, 2016). However, questions and clarifications along the way are always affirmed. If either person feels discomfort, they agree to instantly communicate verbally or non-verbally in a clear manner to "yellow" (slow down or take a pause) or "red" (full stop) the exercise. Consent is revokable at any time from what was opted-into. Nothing is allowed to be added during the session after initial agreement, as a form of practicing respect and fidelity. Hess (CC, 2016) recommends the non-verbal option of "tapping out" with two quick taps to any area or action that is creating discomfort and needs to stop immediately. Never assume that touch done one day will be allowable or desirable the next time. Always negotiate consent and be fully present in the I.N.T.I.M.A.C.Y. of touch.

Touch Training

If a client explicitly consents to touch exercises there are a few steps that currently have been integrated in nurse training (Estabrooks & Morse, 1992) that will help: entering, cueing up, consenting, connection, closure, and appreciation. Entering is the initial pre-touch verbal and somatic implementation of the consent process. The client's self-determination might or might not allow the professional to enter the "bubble" of their personal boundaries. The permeable bubble psychically protects the client from violations. Different areas of the body might have different permeability. Female acculturalized clients might have very little off-limit touch area mapping with trusted professionals (Suvilehto, 2015) due to daily internalizing of unfortunately common misogynistic touch assaults. Male acculturalized clients often have off-limit areas of the pelvic, genital, and buttocks zones for all but partners, friends, and parents. If there is comfort within the clients allowed bubble zone, consent may be negotiated for the specific touch I.N.T.I.M.A.C.Y. While either person may rescind at any time, it is recommended that the professional maintain fidelity and explicitness to the commitment. The professional has explicitly agreed to interact with the client. Connecting is highly nuanced, individual, and complex. It requires vulnerability from both people to share love, care, and kindness. Closure is the conclusion of the touching practice as pre-negotiated, and includes appreciation for the client being open to "bubble bumping" with the professional. It is also a time for mutual reflection and constructive feedback, so that the framework of consent remains a vibrantly updating mutual dialogue.

Touch can balance upon the "resilient edge of resistance" (Mainard; in Jesse, 2020, 46). It should be the "goldilocks" of pressure and duration. If the touch is too soft, it will feel irritating; while if it is too hard, it will feel assaultive. Touch should last enough time to establish firm contact, but not so long that either person feels uncomfortable (Bacorn & Dixon, 1984, 491; in Willison & Masson, 1986). Three to five seconds can be a general timeframe to explore with a client. Routasalo (1999) recommends basic professional training upon 27 areas of touch within most bioscience frameworks: necessary, non-necessary, instrumental, expressive, affectional, procedural, empathic, philanthropic, spontaneous, pragmatic, silent, non-procedural, investigator, therapeutic, systematic, comforting, protective, caring, task, functional, purposeful, connecting, working, orienting, social, work/task, and caring/social touch. Kennedy and Dean (1995) prefer a specifically linear series of touch explorations that can have more erotic potential: hand caress, face caress, foot caress, body image, back caress, front caress, sensual shower, "sexplorations", pleasuring, and intercourse. The beginning of the series can be assisted with a professional, similar to the way that sensate focus can be guided (Masters & Johnson, 1982, 488–489). With initial training and practice, a client can continue through the series solo, with an intimate partner, or a professional with significant additional training. Professionals that are feeling uneasy about a simple hand-to-hand caress should not "level-up" to showering with a client. It is important to know one's personal and professional limits, which is often based upon one's professional training. Basic touch training techniques will be discussed below. Professionals should refer clients to coalition partners that have the requisite training while practicing these training skills. It is better to refer than to create harm.

Practicing Touch

Start somatic exercises with breath awareness, as it helps to quiet the mind, and is a zero-cost tool that people with all bodies can practice anywhere at any time (Hạnh, 1975, 14–22; Zal, 2022). Slowing down the capitalistic sense of urgency is central to sexual mindfulness (Okun, 1999; Proust, 1919, 275–276). The question of "How would you like to be touched?" can be asked days or weeks before any somatic exercise is even considered a possibility. This allows the client time to marinade on what is genuine. Discuss the full intent and "arc" of the somatic treatment plans with the client. This arc must include the ABC's of Awareness, Boundaries, and Communication for consent, safety, and trust (Heartman, 2021). The next increment of treatment might include "May I?" and "Will You?" exercises, but this and no other step along the arc is ever to be expected. The arc might include body acceptance and sexuality education (Dodson, 1974, 57–70; Jesse, 2020, 22). Specific suggestions and somatic practices might guide core erotic issues. And most importantly is a pre-negotiated closure that will be implemented when the client's growth process comes to upeksha (equanimity), a place of harmonious contentment, or an impasse that cannot be professionally resolved.

The "May I/Will You" touch process has a minimum of five reciprocal rounds where the client provides offers of touch and then requests for touch. This is then reciprocated by the professional. Giving the client control of the exercise proactively shifts the power differential by requiring the professional to assume higher potential risk. In the first round, no matter how enticing the offer or request might be, the answer is always "No." This is a way to practice verbalizing and receiving a decline without a sense of identity harm. The second round is also only verbal, but the responses must always be "Yes." There is safety in this step, since both people know that there is zero expectation any touching will occur. Verbalized acceptance of offers or requests, which might differ in actual desires, allows opportunity to discuss traumatogenic fawning patterns of enduring actions not desired. The next two non-touch rounds are similar with a requirement of a "No" and then a "Yes." However, in these two rounds the offers and requests are to be genuinely considered, and both people share their feelings honestly. Each person takes full ownership of their feelings around the affect without judgement. The client is also asked to not internalize any acceptance or rejection of their offers and requests. Playful humor often occurs as the rounds progress and comfort is established. These rounds might be practiced repeatedly across multiple session prior to the next stage where touching is allowed. Start again with the professional assuming higher risk as receiver in the touch exercise. To guide the client, incremental zones between the wrist and up to the elbow; up to the shoulder; hands; arms up to the torso above the clavicle and below the neck; head excluding the face; upper back; lower leg; outer thigh; and lower back. Do not stigmatize or heighten the importance of body zones not yet explored. See Suvilehto (2015) for a visual depiction of the body comfort zones. The genuine comfort of the client's body is to be centered. Ask, don't assume. Awareness of cultural difference is very important to acknowledge and respect. The above body zones can be explored in a linear manner at least three times, and then randomly another five times. Discuss the client's spectrum of apprehension through joy and any particular visceral sensations experienced. When there is comfort, trust, and confidence with these areas additional areas can be explored. Discuss with the client if they would like to progress linearly from the lower back to the belly; neck; face; buttocks; chest; inner thighs; and groin. Unless professionally trained as a surrogate, somatic bodyworker, physical therapist, or similar, it is recommended to remain external of all orifices.

In all of these practice exercises, communication is key. If the client or professional receives an undesired request, they can utilize compassionate Judo. This is a "gentle way" of engaging conflict or potential oppression by re-purposing the inertial energy of the conflict to dissolve into harmony. In the martial arts, it is transmuting the force of someone's attack into defensively flipping the attacker through the air. In sexuality, an example can be shifting someone's request to fuck into sharing quality time and a cup of tea instead. Even when a request is desired, nuanced communication continues to be of the upmost importance with each step of the journey. After all forms of practices, with or without touch, remember the closure step of appreciation, gratitude, and constructive feedback. Have an aftercare plan, so that the professional and client can check-in after a day or two of processing. This will support additional trust, allow the consent framework to continue updating, and help the flow of love.

Conclusion

There are a range of skills and services that have clear client need and can be part of a holistic and collaborative treatment plan. If sexuality professionals cannot role model and guide clients concerning sexual attraction, expectations, boundaries, and consensual touch in the safety of the consultation room, how can clients be expected to be successful in the nuanced complexity of the bedroom?

Four of the policies specifically mandate professionals to proactively seek change of barriers to self-determined client care (ACA, 2014, 8.C; AMA, 2022, IV; ANA, 2015, vii; APA, 1999). This can begin with a simple reflection upon Annon's P.LI.SS.IT. treatment framework (1976). In the current model, Permission (P), Limited Information (LI), and Specific Suggestions (SS) are part of the training of most sexuality healthcare providers. Provision of Intensive Therapy (IT) is reserved for those psychosexually trained and statistically required for less than 18% of clients (ibid.). When a client in a place of low capacity and/or agency receives Permission (P) from a professional for their sexual behavior, attraction, or identity, it can be a positively affirming utilization of power differentials. However, to allow for centralization of self-determination, and a removal of the professional's moral superiority, it is important that the outdated concept of practitioners providing "permission" be removed, and a shift to Acceptance (A) is practiced. Additionally, the integration of a coalition for collaborative and referred treatment has been additionally proposed by Nasserzadeh (2018). A slight restructuring of the "Master's tools" will allow for meta-cognitive reflection prior to any Intensive Therapy. Specialized sexuality professionals do not have the skills to assist every erotic issue, marginalization, or client-centered treatment plan. By shifting Referral (R) from the end to before Intensive Therapy (IT), an opportunity is created for coalition building and collaboration. It also removes the stigma of referral signifying that the professional is lacking or has failed. Asking for help and centering client care demonstrate wisdom. A.LI.SS.R.-IT. can serve as a holistic framework as the sexual revolution continues.

This chapter might inspire the reader to become a Respectful Revolutionary, which is being an agent of change, while being compassionate to people's needs and feelings in the present moment. While striving for change, please concurrently honor that many people feel unease in risking their hegemonic lives by disrupting the status quo or implementing change; no matter how much harm has been experienced or they have been vicariously traumatized. Respectful Revolutionaries critically reflect upon the change that they desire to manifest in the world; and find pathways that are not coercive, forceful, nor perpetuating the harm that wants to be eradicated. Creating coalitions, recognizing what forms of change need to be incremental to allow for cultural inertia, and recognizing what forms of change will only happen when holistic and encompassing many elements of society act swiftly. This is how "we" can be respectful revolutionaries, and how "we" can change the world.

Acknowledgments

Authoring what professionals "should" do is a hypocritical paradox when discussing the falseness of moral superiority. I, the author, was raised in a culture of oppression. While I endeavor to unpack and transgress my own embodied harm to guide future generations, the "language of oppression" (Rich, 1971) are the words I have at this time. Thank you deeply to all of the wise elders that help me continue in learning from a place of imperfection. If this chapter has raised curiosity about the lineage of lateral and transformational thought, please explore: Chuang Tzu; Anne Fausto-Sterling; Audre Lorde; bell hooks; Betty Dodson; Bianca I. Laureano; Brené Brown; Caffyn Jesse; David Bowie; Deconstructivism; Embodiment; Judith Butler; Ken Plummer; Ken Wilber; Lisa Diamond; Lori Brotto; Marcel Proust; Michel Foucault; Paulo Reglus Neves Freire; Phenomenology; Post-Colonial Futurism; Post-Structuralism; Ram Karan Sharma; Jalālal-Dīn Bālkhī Rūmī;

Satya Narayana Goenka; Sen Genshitsu; Stuart Sovatsky; Ted McIlvenna; and Thích Nhất Hạnh. Citations are listed after a few reflective questions.

Questions for Reflection:

1. How would you like to touched?
2. How do you identify personally, professionally, and sexually? Is there a difference between what you present with friends, family, and/or publicly, from what you hold true in your heart?
3. What are your personal values? How do your personal values inform your sense of morality, alignment with societal ethics, and gut feelings about the spectrum of sensuality/sexuality?
4. What are your personal/professional boundaries in providing client care, and how might other professionals supplement your services with their training and offered services?
5. What resources are you willing to contribute (time, money, ideas, labor, reputation) to locally, regionally, or internationally risk supporting holistic client-centered warmth, caring relationships, touch, and love?

References

Attwood, Feona. (2007). Sluts and Riot Grrrls: Female Identity and Sexual Agency. *Journal of Gender Studies, 16*(3), pp. 233–247; DOI: 10.1080/09589230701562921

Annon, Jack S. (1976). The PLISSIT Model: A Proposed Conceptual Scheme for the Behavioral Treatment of Sexual Problems. *Journal of Sex Education and Therapy, 2*(1), 1–15; DOI: 10.1080/01614576.1976.11074483

Bacorn, Christopher N.; & Dixon, David N. (1984). The effects of touch on depressed and vocationally undecided clients. *Journal of Counseling Psychology, 31*(4), p.488–496; DOI: 10.1037/0022-0167.31.4.488

Barnett, Jeffrey E.; Behnke, Stephen H.; Rosenthal, Susan L; & Koocher, Gerald P. (2007). In Case of Ethical Dilemma, Break Glass: Commentary on Ethical Decision Making in Practice. American Psychological Association; *Professional Psychology: Research and Practice, 38*(1), pp.7–12; DOI: 10.1037/0735-7028.38.1.7

Barker, Chris; & Jane, Emma. (2016). *Cultural Studies: Theory and Practice.* 5th Ed; Sage Publications.

Baudrillard, Jean. (1981/1994). *Simulacra and Simulation.* University of Michigan Press; ISBN: 978-0472065219

Beauchamp, Tom L.; & Childress, James F. (1979). *Principles of Biomedical Ethics.* Oxford University Press; ISBN: 978-0195024876

Beauchamp, Tom L.; & Childress, James F. (2019). *Principles of Biomedical Ethics.* Oxford University Press; ISBN: 978-0190640873

Binik, Yitzchak M.; & Meana, Marta. (2009). The Future of Sex Therapy: Specialization or Marginalization? *Archives of Sexual Behavior, 38,* pp.1016–1027; DOI: 10.1007/s10508-009-9475-9

Bjorbækmo, Wenche Schrøder; & Mengshoel, Anne Marit. (2016). A Touch of Physiotherapy: The Significance and Meaning of Touch in the Practice of Physiotherapy. *Physiotherapy Theory and Practice*, pp.1–10; DOI: 10.3109/09593985.2015.1071449

Bolelli, Murat. (2019). The Effects of Dark Triad (Machiavellianism, Narcissism, Psychopathy) on the Love Attitudes. *Journal of Current Debates in Social Sciences*, 2(2), pp.164–173.; DOI: 10.37154/ijopec.2019.3

Brotto, Lori.; Krychman, Michael.; & Jacobson, Pamela. (2008). Eastern Approaches for Enhancing Women's Sexuality: Mindfulness, Acupuncture, and Yoga. *Journal of Sexual Medicine*, 5, pp.2,741–2,748.

Brown, Brené (2013). *The Power of Vulnerability*. Sounds True; ASIN: B00D1Z9RFU.

Brown, Robert D.; & Newman, Dianna, L. (1992). Ethical Principles and Evaluation Standards: Do they match? *Evaluation Review*, 16(6), pp.650–663; DOI: 10.1177/0193841X9201600605

Butler, Judith. (2004). *Undoing Gender*. Routledge; ISBN: 978-0415969239

Chiang, Howard. (2018). Introduction: Writing the History of Sexuality in China. pp.3–15; in Chiang, Howard. *Sexuality in China: Histories of Power and Pleasure*. University of Washington Press; ISBN: 978-0295743479

Combahee River Collective. (1977/1979). A Black Feminist Statement. pp.210–218; in Eisenstein, Zillah R. *Capitalist Patriarchy and the Case for Socialist Feminism*. Monthly Review Press; ISBN: 978-0853454762

Czimbal, Bob; & Zadikov, Maggie. (1991). *A Guide to Healthy Touch: Vitamin T*. Open Book Publishers; ISBN: 1-878793-00-4

DeBeauvoir, Simone. (1953/1956). *The Second Sex*. Jonathan Cape; ISBN: 978-0679724513

Demos, John. (2008). *The Enemy Within: 2000 Years of Witch-Hunting in the Western World*. Viking; ISBN: 978-0670019991

Diamond, Lisa M. (2009). *Sexual Fluidity: Understanding Women's Love and Desire*. Harvard University Press; ISBN: 978-0674032262

Dodson, Betty. (1974/1996). *Sex for One: The Joy of Selfloving*. Three Rivers Press; ISBN: 0-517-86607-3

Drescher, Jack. (2013). Ghosts in the Consulting Room: A Discussion of Anson's 'Ghosts in the Dressing Room'. *Journal of Gay & Lesbian Mental Health*, 17(1), pp.112–120; DOI: 10.1080/19359705.2013.740658

Ehrenreich, Barbara; & English, Deirdre. (2010). *Witches, Midwives, & Nurses: A History of Women Healers*. Feminist Press; ISBN: 978-1558616615

Equicola, Mario. (1525/1989) *De natura d'amore* (*On the Nature of Love*). libro quarto; Capelli; ASIN: B00KXARQ0Y

Erel, Umut; Haritaworn, Lin; et.al. (2010). On the Depoliticisation of Intersectionality Talk: Conceptualising Multiple Oppressions in Critical Sexuality Studies; in Taylor, Yvette; Hines, Sally; & Casey, Mark. *Theorizing Intersectionality and Sexuality. Genders and Sexualities in the Social Sciences*. Palgrave Macmillan, London; pp.56–73; DOI: 10.1057/9780230304093_4

Estabrooks, C. A.; & Morse, J. M. (1992). Toward a Theory of Touch: The Touching Process and Acquiring a Touching Style. *Journal of Advanced Nursing*, 17(4), pp.448–456; DOI: 10.1111/j.1365-2648.1992.tb01929.x

Farley, Margaret. (2006). *Just Love: A Framework for Christian Sexual Ethics*. Continuum; ISBN: 978-0826429247

Fausto-Sterling, Anne. (2012). *Sex/Gender: Biology in a Social World*. Routledge; ISBN: 978-0415881463

Ferenczi, Sándor. (1949/1988). Confusion of the Tongues Between the Adults and the Child: The Language of Tenderness and of Passion. *International Journal of Psycho-Analysis, 30*, 225–230; in *Contemporary Psychoanalysis, 24*(2), 196–206. DOI: 10.1080/00107530.1988.10746234

Ferrer, Jorge N. (2021). *Love and Freedom: Transcending Monogamy and Polyamory (Diverse Sexualities, Genders, and Relationships)*. Rowman & Littlefield Publishers; ISBN: 978-1538156575

Fine, Michelle; & McClelland, Sara. (2006). Sexuality Education and Desire: Still Missing after All These Years. *Harvard Educational Review, 76*(3), 297–338; DOI: 10.17763/haer.76.3.w5042g23122n6703

Fiske, Susan T.; Cuddy, Amy J. C.; Glick, Peter. (2006). Universal Dimensions of Social Cognition: Warmth and Competence. *TRENDS in Cognitive Sciences, 11*(2), 77–83; DOI: 10.1016/j.tics.2006.11.005

Foucault, Michel. (1961). *Madness & Civilization*. Librairie Plon; ISBN: 0-679-72110-X.

Foucault, Michel. (1978/1980). *The History of Sexuality: Volume I, An Introduction*. Vintage Books; ISBN: 978-0394740263

Freire, Paulo Reglus Neves. (1970/2000). *Pedagogy of the Oppressed*. Penguin Random House; ISBN: 0-8264-1276-9

Freire, Paulo Reglus Neves. (1978/1983). *Pedagogy in Process: The Letters to Guinea-Bissau*. Continuum; ISBN: 0-8264-0136-8

Gagnon, John; & Simon, William. (1973). The Social Origins of Sexual Development; in Gagnon, John; & Simon, William. (2005). *Sexual Conduct: The Social Sources of Human Sexuality*. Aldine Transaction; pp.1–19.

Goenka, Satya Narayan. (2004). *Guidelines for Practicing Vipassana Meditation*. Vipassana Research Institute.

Gottlieb, M. C. (1993). Avoiding Exploitive Dual Relationships: A Decision-making Model. *Psychotherapy: Theory, Research, Practice, Training, 30*(1), 41–48; DOI: 10.1037/0033-3204.30.1.41

Habermas, Jürgen. (1990). Morality, Society and Ethics: An Interview with Torben Hviid Nielsen. *Acta Sociologica, 33*(2), 93–114; DOI: 10.1177/000169939003300201

Hạnh, Thich Nhất. (1975/1999). *The Miracle of Mindfulness: An Introduction to the Practice of Meditation*. Beacon Press; ISBN: 978-0807012390

Harcourt, Christine; & Donovan, Basil. (2005). The Many Faces of Sex Work. *Sexually Transmitted Infections, 81*(3), 201–206. DOI: 10.1136/sti.2004.012468

Harlow, Harry F. (1958). The Nature of Love. *American Psychologist, 13*(12), 673–685; DOI: 10.1037/h0047884

Harris, Kamala; Nhu, T. T. (1997). Sex Surrogate Says Her Mission is to Help the Dysfunctional. *San Jose Mercury News*; 4 October 1997, 7A.

Harrison, Carmel; Jones, Robert S. P.; & Huws, Jaci C. (2012). We're People who Don't Touch: Exploring Clinical Psychologists' Perspectives on their Use of Touch in Therapy. *Counselling Psychology Quarterly, 25*(3), 277–287, DOI: 10.1080/09515070.2012.671595

Hawai'i. (1996). *Aloha Spirit*; Revised Statutes §5-7.5.

Heartman, Andrew. (2021). Collaborating w/Surrogate Partners in the Triadic Model; [Webinar].

Hippocrates. (447BCE). *Hippocratic Oath*.

hooks, bell. (1984/1994). *Teaching to Transgress: Education as the Practice of Freedom*. Routledge; ISBN-13: 978-0415908085

Houser, Rick; Wilczenski, Felicia L.; & Ham, MaryAnna. (2006). *Culturally Relevant Ethical Decision Making in Counseling.* Sage Publications; ISBN: 1-4129-0587-7

Hume, David. (1740/1986). *A Treatise of Human Nature: Being an Attempt to Introduce the Experimental Method of Reasoning into Moral Subjects.* Penguin Classics; ISBN: 978-0140432442

Irvine, Janice M. (2014). Is Sexuality Research 'Dirty Work'? Institutionalized Stigma in the Production of Sexual Knowledge. *Sexualities, 17*(5/6), 632–656; DOI: 10.1177/1363460713516338

Irvine, Janice M. (2015). The Other Sex Work: Stigma in Sexuality Research. *Social Currents, 2*(2), 116–125; DOI: 10.1177/2329496515579762

Jackson, Helen Hunt. (1881/2003). *A Century of Dishonor: A Sketch of the United States Government's Dealings with Some of the Indian Tribes.* Harper & Brothers; Dover Publications; ISBN: 978-0486426983.

Jesse, Caffyn. (2020). *Intimacy Educator: Teaching through Touch.* EcoSpirit; ISBN: 979–8623507136

Jones, Irma S.; Rivas, Olivia; & Mancillas, Margarita. (2009). A Model for Teaching Ethical Meta-Principles: A Descriptive Experience. *Journal of Instructional Pedagogies, 10*, 30–39.

Kant, Immanuel. (1785/2020). *Groundwork of the Metaphysics of Morals.* Oxford University Press; ISBN: 978-0198786191

Kant, Immanuel. (1788/2004). *Critique of Practical Reason.* Dover Publications; ISBN: 978-0486434452

Kant, Immanuel. (1797/1991). *The Metaphysics of Morals.* Cambridge University Press; ISBN: 978-0521316576

Kasai, Makiko. (2009). The Role of Japanese Culture in Psychological Health: Implications for Counseling and Clinical Psychology. pp.159–170; in Gerstein, Lawrence H.; Heppner, P. P.; Ægisdóttir, Stefanía; Leung, Seung-Ming Alvin; & Norsworthy, Kathryn L. *International Handbook of Cross-Cultural Counseling: Cultural Assumptions and Practices Worldwide.* Sage Publishing; ISBN: 978-1412959568

Kaufman, Scott B. (2019). The Light Triad vs. Dark Triad of Personality. *Scientific American, 30*(2), 19.

Kennedy, Adele P.; & Dean, Susan. (1995). *Touching for Pleasure.* Chatsworth Press; ISBN: 978-0917181115

Kirschner, Andrew S. (2005). *Back Together: Hands-On Healing for Couples.* Running Press; ISBN: 978-0762424030

Kitchener, Karen S. (1984). Intuition, Critical Evaluation, and Ethical Principles: The Foundation for Ethical Decisions in Counseling Psychology. *Counseling Psychologist, 12*, 43–55; DOI: 10.1177/0011000084123005

Kitchener, Karen S. (1996). There is More to Ethics than Principles. *Counseling Psychologist, 24*, 92–97.; DOI: 10.1177/0011000096241005

Kohlberg, Lawrence; Levine, Charles; & Hewer, Alexandra. (1983). Moral Stages: A Current Formulation and a Response to Critics; in Meacham, J. A. *Contributions to Human Development*; v.10, Karger; ISBN: 978-3805537162

Kohlberg, Lawrence. (1973). The Claim to Moral Adequacy of a Highest Stage of Moral Judgment. *Journal of Philosophy, 70*(18), 630; DOI: 10.2307/2025030

Koltko-Rivera, Mark E. (2004). The Psychology of Worldviews. *Review of General Psychology, 8*(1), 3–58; DOI: 10.1037/1089-2680.8.1.3

Kosierb, Samantha; & Bilodeau, Cynthia. (2020). Supervising the Use of Touch: A Phenomenological Study. *Body, Movement and Dance in Psychotherapy*, 1–15; DOI: 10.1080/17432979.2020.1787517

Laureano, Bianca Ivette; & Flowers, Sara C. (2018). Writing Ourselves into Existence: Healing Through Collaborative Curriculum Development. *Journal of Critical Thought and Praxis*, 7(2), 50–60.

Le, Thao N.; & Jackman, Teneya. (2022). Beyond Aloha: Can University of Hawai'i Students Cultivate Native Hawaiian Relational Awareness in a Mindfulness Course, ch.1, pp.3–17; in Fleming, Crystal M.; Womack, Veronica Y.; & Proulx, Jeffrey. *Beyond White Mindfulness: Critical Perspectives on Racism, Well-being and Liberation*. Routledge; ISBN: 978-0367548629; DOI: 10.4324/9781003090922-2

Lee, John Alan. (1977). A Typology of Styles of Loving. *Personality and Social Psychology Bulletin*, 3(2), 173–182. DOI: 10.1177/014616727700300204

Lorde, Audre. (1979). The Master's Tools Will Never Dismantle the Master's House; New York University, Institute for the Humanities; in *Sister Outsider: Essays and Speeches*. pp.110–113; Crossing Press; ISBN: 978-1580911863

Luke (85) Gospel According to Luke; in Campbell, Gordon. (1611/2010). *The Holy Bible*: King James *Version*. Oxford University Press; ISBN: 978-0199557608

MacFarlane, Rachel T.; Fuller, Celene; Wakefield, Chris; & Brents, Barbara G. (2017). Sex Industry and Sex Workers in Nevada. *Social Health of Nevada: Leading Indicators and Quality of Life in the Silver State*. University of Nevada, pp.1–38.

McIntosh, Peggy. (1988). White Privilege and Male Privilege: A Personal Account of Coming to See Correspondences Through Work in Women's Studies; Working Paper 189; Wellesley College, Centers for Women.

Marcia, James. (1966). Development and Validity of Ego-Identity Status. *Journal of Personality and Social Psychology*, 3(5), 551–558; DOI: 10.1037/h0023281

Masters, William H.; Johnson, Virginia E; & Kolodny, Robert C. (1977). *Ethical Issues in Sex Therapy and Research*. Little Brown & Co.; ISBN: 0-316-549-835

Masters, William; Johnson, Virginia; and Kolodny, Robert. (1982/1986). *On Sex and Human Loving*. Little Brown and Company; ISBN: 0-316-54998-3

McIlvenna, Ted; Ayres, Tony; Lyon, Phyllis; Myers, Frank; Rila, Margo; Rubenstein, Maggi; Smith, Carolyn; & Sutton, Laird. (1975). *Sexual Attitude Restructuring SARguide for a Better Sex Life: A Self-Help Program for Personal Sexual Enrichment/Education*. National Sex Forum; ISBN: 9780913566015

McIlvenna, Ted; & Sutton, Laird. (1977). *Meditations on the Gift of Sexuality*. Specific Press; ISBN: 0-930846-01-X

Merleau-Ponty, Maurice. (1945/2002). *Phenomenology of Perception*. Routledge; ISBN: 978-0415278409

Mezirow, Jack. (1997). Transformative Learning: Theory to Practice. *New Directions for Adult and Continuing Education*, 74, 5–12; Jossey-Bass Publishers; DOI: 10.1002/ace.7401

Moulton, Ian Frederick. (2010). In Praise of Touch: Mario Equicola and the Nature of Love. *Senses & Society*, 5(1), 119–130; DOI: 10.2752/174589310X12549020528338

Nasserzadeh, Sara. (2018). Practical Recommendations to Work with Couples presenting with 'Unconsummated Marriages' in Any Health Care Settings.

Nelson, Melissa K. (2017). Getting Dirty: The Eco-Eroticism of Women in Indigenous Oral Literatures, ch.7, pp.229–260; in Barker, Joanne. *Critically Sovereign: Indigenous Gender, Sexuality, and Feminist Studies*. Duke University Press; ISBN: 978-0822363651; DOI: 10.1215/9780822373162-008

Nzegwu, Nkiru. (2011). Ósunality (or African Eroticism); in Tamale, Sylvia. (2011). *African Sexualities: A Reader*. Pambazuka Press; pp.253–270; ISBN: 978-0857490162

Okun, Tema. (1999). *White Supremacy Culture*. dRworks.

Owen, Pamela M.; & Gillentine, Jonathan. (2011). Please Touch the Children: Appropriate Touch in the Primary Classroom. *Early Child Development and Care, 181*(6), 857–868; DOI: 10.1080/03004430.2010.497207

Paulhus, Delroy L.; & Williams, Kevin M. (2002). The Dark Triad of Personality: Narcissism, Machiavellianism and Psychopathy. *Journal of Research in Personality, 36*(6), 556–563; DOI: 10.1016/S0092-6566(02)00505-6

Perel, Esther. (2017). *Mating in Captivity: Reconciling the Erotic + the Domestic.* Harper Paperbacks; chs1–4; ISBN: 978-0060753641

Piaget, Jean. (1932). *The Moral Judgment of the Child.* Routledge & Kegan Paul; ISBN: 9780415849623

Plummer, Ken. (2012). Critical Sexuality Studies, pp.243–268; in Ritzer, George. *Companion to Sociology*. Wiley-Blackwell; ISBN: 978-1444330397

Plummer, Kenneth. (1975). *Sexual Stigma: An Interactionist Account.* Routledge Kegan & Paul; ISBN: 978-0710080608

Proust, Marcel. (1919/1965). Sunday the 2nd of March: Dinner at the Ritz Hotel; in Nicolson, Harold G. *Peacemaking 1919: Being Reminiscences of the Paris Peace Conference; Grosset & Dunlap.* ASIN: B000K0J2WC; Simon Publications; ISBN: 978-1931541541

Punzo, Vincent A.; & Meara, Naomi M. (1993). The Virtues of a Psychology of Personal Morality. *Journal of Theoretical & Philosophical Psychology, 13*(1), 25–39; DOI: 10.1037/h0091117

Queen, Carol. (1997). Sex radical politics, sex-positive feminist thought, and whore stigma, pp.125–135; in Nagle, Jill. *"Whores and Other Feminists".* Routledge; ISBN 978-0415918220

Queen, Carol. (2014). What Sex-Positivity Is, And Is Not; [Weblog].

Retsas, Spyros. (2019). First Do No Harm: The Impossible Oath, Rapid Response. *British Medical Journal, 366*(l4734), rr2; [DOI]: 10.1136/bmj.l4734

Rich, Adrienne. (1971). *The Will to Change: Poems* 1968-1970. p.15; W. W. Norton & Company; ISBN: 978-0393043617

Rorty, Richard. (1991). Feminism and Pragmatism. *Radical Philosophy, 59*, 3–14; DOI: 10.4324/9781003061502-10

Routasalo, Pirkko. (1999). Physical Touch in Nursing Studies: A Literature Review. *Journal of Advanced Nursing, 30*(4), 843–850. DOI: 10.1046/j.1365-2648.1999.01156.x

Rubin, Gayle S. (1984). Thinking Sex: Notes for a Radical Theory of the Politics of Sexuality, pp.267–319; in Vance, C. S. *Pleasure and Danger: Exploring Female Sexuality.* Routledge; ISBN: 978 0710202482; DOI: 10.4324/9780203966105-21

Rubin, Gayle S. (2011). Blood under the bridge: Reflections on Thinking sex. *GLQ: A Journal of Lesbian and Gay Studies, 17*(1), 15–48; DOI: 10.1215/10642684-2010-015

Rūmī, Jalālal-Dīn Bālkhī. (1244/1995). *The Essential Rūmī.* Harper; ISBN: 0-06-250958-6.

Schermer Seller, Tina. (2017). *Sex, God & the Conservative Church: Erasing Shame from Sexual Intimacy.* Routledge; ISBN: 978-1138674981

Schiller, Patricia. (1973/1977). *Creative Approach to Sex Education and Counseling.* Associate Press; IBSN: 0-8096-1923-7

Sen Genshitsu. (1980/1996). *Urasenke Chanoyu.* Handbook Two, Urasenke Foundation Publications; ASIN: B000UV0D3I

Sharma, Ram Karan; Pitts, Carol; & Morgan, Les. (2015). *Bhagavadgita.* CreateSpace Independent Publishing Platform; ISBN: 978–1466269958

Sovatsky, Stuart. (1999). *Eros, Consciousness, and Kundalini: Deepening Sensuality through Tantric Celibacy and Spiritual Intimacy.* Park Street Press; ISBN: 978–0892818303.

Stanger, Elle. (2017). I'm a Sex Worker Who Is Sick of Female Misogyny. Huffington Post.

Stayton, William R. (1992). Conflicts in Crisis; Effects of Religious Belief Systems on Sexual Health, pp.203–218; in Green, Ronald. *Religion and Sexual Health.* Kluwer Academic Publishers; ISBN: 978-9401579643

Stayton, William R. (2002). A Theology of Sexual Pleasure; SIECUS Report, 30(4), 27–29.

Suvilehto, Juulia T.; Glerean, Enrico; Dunbar, Robin I. M.; Hari, Riitta; & Nummenmaa, Lauri. (2015). Topography of Social Touching Depends on Emotional Bonds Between Humans. *Proceedings of the National Academy of Sciences*; DOI: 10.1073/pnas.1519231112

Swan, Tracy A. (2002). COMING OUT AND SELFDISCLOSURE: Exploring the Pedagogical Significance in Teaching Social Work Students about Homophobia and Heterosexism. Canadian Association for Social Work Education (CASWE), *Canadian Social Work Review*, 19(1), 5–23; JSTOR: 41669744

Takacs, David. (2003). How Does Your Positionality Bias Your Epistemology? *The NEA Higher Education Journal: Thought & Action*, 27–38.

Tamale, Sylvia. (2011). *African Sexualities: A Reader.* Pambazuka Press; ISBN: 978-0857490162

Tario, Josue. (2019). Critical Spirituality: Decolonizing the Self, pp.179–193; in Wane, N. N. *Decolonizing the Spirit in Education and Beyond: Spirituality, Religion, and Education*; DOI: 10.1007/978-3-030-25320-2_12

Thwaites, Rachel. (2017). Making a Choice or Taking a Stand? Choice Feminism, Political Engagement and the Contemporary Feminist Movement. *Feminist Theory*, 18(1), 55–68; DOI: 10.1177/1464700116683657

Tiziano, Shay; & Tiziano, Stefanos. (2021). *Creating Captivating Classes: A Guide for Kink, Sexuality, and Relationship Presenters.* Twisted Windows; ISBN: 978–0578942247

Tolman, Deborah; Bowman, Christin; & Fahs, Breanne. (2014). Sexuality and Embodiment, chp.25; in Tolman, Deborah; & Diamond, Lisa. *APA Handbook of Sexuality and Psychology*; *v1, Person-Based Approaches*. American Psychological Association; DOI: 10.1037/14193-025

Tsai; Daniel Fu-Chang. (1999). Ancient Chinese Medical Ethics and the Four Principles of Biomedical Ethics. *Journal of Medical Ethics*, 25, 315–321; DOI: 10.1136/jme.25.4.315

Tune, David. (2001). Is Touch a Valid Therapeutic Intervention? Early Returns from a Qualitative Study of Therapists' Views. *Counselling and Psychotherapy Research: Linking Research with Practice*, 1(3), 167–171, DOI: 10.1080/14733140112331385020

Twigg, Julia; Wolkowitz, Carol; Cohen, Rachel Lara; & Nettleton, Sarah. (2011). Conceptualising Body Work in Health and Social Care. *Sociology of Health & Illness*, 33(2), 171–188; DOI: 10.1111/j.1467-9566.2010.01323.x

Tzu, Chuang. (280BCE/1974). *Inner Chapters.* Vintage Publishers; ISBN: 978-0394719900

UUA - Unitarian Universalist Association. (2021). Planning Guide for Our Whole Lives / Sexuality and Our Faith Facilitator Trainings; [Training Manual].

Urofsky, Robert I.; Engels, Dennis W.; & Engebretson, Ken. (2008). Kitchener's Principle Ethics: Implications for Counseling Practice and Research. *Counseling and Values*, *53*, 67–78; DOI: 10.1002/j.2161-007X.2009.tb00114.x

von Krafft-Ebing, Richard Freiherr. (1886/1998). *Psychopathia Sexualis: Eine Klinisch-Forensische Studie (Sexual Psychopathy: A Clinical-Forensic Study)*. Verlag von Ferdinand Enke; Arcade Publishing; ISBN: 978-1559704267

Wilber, Ken. (2001). *No Boundary Eastern and Western Approaches to Personal Growth*. Witness Exercise, Shambhala Press, pp.128–132; ISBN: 978-1570627439

Williams, Simon; & Bendelow, Gillian. (1998). The Lived Body. in *The Lived Body: Sociological Themes, Embodied Issues*. Routledge; ISBN: 0-415-19426-1.

Willison, Beverly G.; & Masson, Robert L. (1986). The Role of Touch in Therapy: An Adjunct to Communication. *Journal of Counseling & Development*, *64*(8), 497–500; DOI: 10.1002/j.1556-6676.1986.tb01180.x

Wiseman, Howard. (2008). The Roman Empire: 18 Centuries in 19 Maps. in Halsall, Guy. *Barbarian Migrations and the Roman West*, 376–568. Cambridge University Press; ISBN: 978-0521435437

Yarber, William; & Sayad, Barbara. (2010). Sexuality Education for Youth in the United States: Conflict, Content, Research and Recommendation. *Kwartalnik Pedagogiczny*, *2*(216), 147–162.

Zal, Fredrick. (2022 scheduled). Sexual Mindfulness: Lineage & Practice Techniques. *Journal of Sexual Medicine* Review.

Zal, Fredrick. (2019/2022). Consent Basics. Consent Academy; [Webinar].

Zhang, Daquing; & Cheng, Zhifan. (2000). Medicine is a Humane Art: The Basic Principles of Professional Ethics in Chinese Medicine. *Hastings Center Report*, *30*(4), 8–12; DOI: 10.2307/3527656

Policy Reviewed:

AAMFT - American Association for Marriage and Family Therapy. (2015). Code of Ethics.

AANP - American Association of Naturopathic Physicians. (2015). Code of Ethics.

AASECT - American Association of Sexuality Educators Counselors & Therapists. (2014). Position on Touch and the AASECT Certified Professional.

AASECT - American Association of Sexuality Educators Counselors & Therapists. (2014.ccc). Code of Ethics & Conduct for AASECT Certified Members.

AASECT - American Association of Sexuality Educators Counselors & Therapists. (2019.pg). Presenter Guidelines for AASECT Presentations that Include Live Demonstrations.

AASECT - American Association of Sexuality Educators Counselors & Therapists. (2022.cst). AASECT Certification Application: Sex Therapist.

AASECT - American Association of Sexuality Educators Counselors & Therapists. (2022.csc). AASECT Certification Application: Sexuality Counselor.

AASECT - American Association of Sexuality Educators Counselors & Therapists. (2022.cse). AASECT Certification Application: Sexuality Educator.

ACA - American Counseling Association. (2014). Code of Ethics.

ACOG - American College of Obstetricians and Gynecologists. (2018). Code of Professional Ethics.

ACSB - Association of Certified Sexological Bodyworkers. (2014). Code of Professional Conduct and Ethics.

AMA - American Medical Association. (2022). Code of Medical Ethics.

AMTA - American Massage Therapy Association. (2010). Code of Ethics.

ANA - American Nursing Association. (2015). *Code of Ethics for Nurses with Interpretive Statements.* ISBN: 978-1558105997.

AOA - American Osteopathic Association. (2016). Code of Ethics.

AOA - American Osteopathic Association. (2022) "Proposed Amendments to the AOA Code of Ethics".

APA - American Psychological Association. (2018). Introduction: Feminist Therapy— Not for Cisgender Women Only; in Brown, Laura S. *Feminist Therapy*. American Psychological Association; ISBN: 978-1433829116; DOI: 10.1037/0000092-001

APA - American Psychological Association. (2017). Ethical Principles of Psychologists and Code of Conduct.

APA - American Psychological Association. (1999). Feminist Therapy Institute Code of Ethics' Adapted from (1996) The Feminist Therapy Institute Code of Ethics; Feminist Therapy Institute. *Women & Therapy*, 19, 79–91.

APTA – American Physical Therapy Association. (2010). Code of Ethics for the Physical Therapist.

AUA - American Urological Association. (2004). Code of Ethics.

BACP - British Association for Counselling and Psychotherapy. (2018). Ethical Framework for the Counselling Professions.

CC – Certified Cuddler: Hess, Samantha. (2016). Certified Cuddler Rules.

DomCon. (2021). Privacy Policy, Terms of Service, Terms and Conditions.

IPSA - International Professional Surrogates Association. (2020.ce). Code of Ethics.

IPSA - International Professional Surrogates Association. (2020.ls). Legal and Ethical Status.

KECC Collective. (2019/2021). Kink Education Code of Conduct, pp.423–435; in Tiziano, Shay; & Tiziano, Stefanos. *Creating Captivating Classes: A Guide for Kink, Sexuality, and Relationship Presenters.* Twisted Windows; ISBN: 978-0578942247

NASW - National Association of Social Workers. (2021). Code of Ethics of the National Association of Social Workers.

NCBTMB - National Certification Board for Therapeutic Massage & Bodywork. (2017). Code of Ethics.

SPC - Surrogate Partner Collective. (2022.el). Surrogate Partner Therapy in the United States: Ethical and Legal.

SPC - Surrogate Partner Collective. (2022.sc). Surrogate Partner Code of Conduct.

SPC - Surrogate Partner Collective. (2022.cc). Clinician Code of Conduct.

SWAN - Sex Workers' Rights Advocacy Network. (2021). Sex Work and Feminism: A Guide on the Feminist Principles of Sex Worker Organizing.

TCA - Therapist Certification Association. (2015). Code of Ethical and Professional Conduct.

YJ - Yoga Journal; Barrett, Jennifer. (2007). The Trouble with Touch. *Yoga Journal*, 33(4).

YJ - Yoga Journal; Cohen, Michael H. (2007). The Ethics and Liabilities of Touch. *Yoga Journal*, 33(4).

YJ - Yoga Journal; Siber, Kate. (2015). Everything You Need to Know About the Yamas and Niyamas. *Yoga Journal*, 41(5).

5 Allyship

From Passion to Influence

Chasity Fowlkes

Growing up in a small rural town causes one to dream big. One may have aspirations in life that most cannot fathom or have a drive and work ethic that supports it. I can honestly say that this plays a massive part about why I work and grind so hard and pursue every dream I've had. What I mean is sleepless nights, juggling multiple jobs and projects, sacrificing time with my children, or things that I wanted to do in order to accomplish what was necessary to get to where I wanted to be. I strive to show my children that they can achieve whatever they put their mind to no matter the circumstances.

Being a professional in the sexuality field comes with its set of judgments and misconceptions. To be a black sexuality professional is a whole different ball game. As a Licensed Mental Health Counselor, I have to deal with many biases, prejudices, and roadblocks due to my skin color and the foundation that created my field. These experiences have caused me and many others to have to work twice as hard, twice as long, and still not be able to have the same opportunities. I've always taken the stance that I can either complain about my life, or I can do something to change it. So, this is what I did.

I've always been very sexually open-minded and curious about things that most people outside of the sexual health field find taboo, and this started when I was a young girl who found and watched my mother's porn. I cannot remember my physiological response, but I remember enjoying watching it. I also wonder if there may have been some internal struggle with that enjoyment since I was sexually abused by a relative of my sister's. I didn't share this with anyone until I was an adult and in my Master's program due to the stigma and not fully understanding what was happening when I was younger. Through the cards that I was dealt growing up, I determined that I would want to be able to show people that even when bad things happen to me/them sexually, it doesn't have to be or change my/their identity. I still deserve pleasure; I can have a fulfilling sex life, and sensuality can be a safe way to show intimacy.

This proclamation was my initial interest in this field of sexuality. I began hosting in-home adult parties as a young adult between the age of 18 and 19 with a fantastic rep from The Pleasure Company. I met her because I would have ladies' nights and co-ed parties. The licking, blowing, and touching

DOI: 10.4324/9781003314660-5

ignited happiness and excitement within those who were partnered and non-partnered. The rep eventually talked me into becoming a rep myself. I thoroughly enjoyed it. Educating people who predominantly looked like me in a fun and interactive way that sex was not taboo or a "nasty thing" but that it was natural, normal, and a part of life that meant so much. Their feedback from the parties and reviews of their experience implementing the tips and using the toys was such powerful reassurance that I chose the right direction. Getting involved in this business was easy. It was a multi-level marketing company that required a low start up cost and low to no monthly maintenance cost I kept inventory on hand, but it didn't require a large investment. There was absolutely no engagement in sexual activity of any sort and there were many professional boundaries that were set that made this process one that was both pleasant and enjoyable. There was no real need for marketing as you are automatically listed on the company's website and the rest of your business came from word-of-mouth from the family and friends of those who had thrown parties with you before.

Although I loved educating and entertaining people about sexual and sensual things, it was a real-life tragedy in my now ex-husband's family that led me to see that my dream to become a lawyer may not be the correct path. My desire to help others was solid and apparent, but I decided that I would do so as a Licensed Clinical Psychologist or therapist.

For as long as I can remember, I have been very open and outspoken about the things that were important to me. My grandma, Mae, always reminded me that when I was two years old, I told her, "I think I was born to talk." Talking is a huge part of what a creative coach, visionary, and CEO do, but listening is also essential. While working on my Master's degree in Counseling, one of my professors suggested that I watch Barbara Walter's *Twenty-Twenty* special about transgender youth. I remember watching this and truly being touched by all the stories of the trans children and their families as they moved toward transitioning socially and medically. Jazz Jennings, a now transgender activist and reality TV star was maybe four years old in this episode. She had such an opening, vulnerable, and touching conversation about how she saw herself as a mermaid. She possessed the level of certainty in her own identity, along with the determination of her family to listen to her voice and seek professional help and guidance. Her family did so while making the world as safe as possible for their trans daughter, making it clear to me that this population was whom I am called to assist.

My focus from that point on has been to learn as much as possible to better assist those within the LGBTQ+ community. That was the point in my career when I decided to become a Certified Sex Therapist. I understood that getting my MA in Counseling was a significant step to clinically helping others. Still, I also understood that this level of education would not put me in a position to truly get the skills and tools I needed to assist those I had decided to focus on helping. I also understood that this would come with a hefty price tag. Most of the programs cost upward of $7,500–$11,000 for your AASECT Certification. It is definitely an investment and most either take out private loans or pay out of their pockets, as there is no Pell grant and scholarships are few and far between. I initially planned on attending Dr. Lee's school after talking to her over the phone, but that didn't happen as I was pregnant with my third child and I put Sex Therapy School on hold.

Fast forward a few years following my divorce, I began my journey to become a Certified Sex Therapist. It was a huge financial sacrifice and took much time to complete as a single mother working full time. However, I knew that it would pay off in the long run. I'm able to do the work that I love and I'm passionate about with the people that I chose to lend my expertise to. In other words, I get paid to talk to people about relationships and sex. What happened during my time in sex therapy school was a bit shocking. I'm not sure why, but not having instructors who looked like me was the norm. The fact that I completed the school and education and didn't learn how to do this vital work with people that looked like me rattled me. Before finishing school, I reached out to someone I looked up to, Dr. James Wadley, and I had a short, candid conversation. I asked, "Why do we not have sex therapy schools with instructors who look like us. Why are we not getting any of these coins?" He told me these exact words "I don't know, sis, but if you create it, I will help."

When there are no safe and qualified spaces to help us on this journey, *we can create them.* We being people of color and those who racialized or Indigenous.

I reached out again in 2018 and held him to it. I began to think of the most influential people in my life that I could trust with a project of this magnitude and those who work I adored within the black sexuality field. I call this group of people the Dream Team. They serve as the Advisory Board. In 2019, the National Institute for Sexual Health & Wellness became an official entity and a CE provider for AASECT, the American Association for Sexuality Educators, Counselors and Therapists. Outlining the business plan and setting up the final budget was by far the most difficult part of the process. When you want the best, you have to make sure that you can pay them. My original vision for NISHW was to create a table that would allow others to both have a seat and create additional streams of income for those who look like me. Projected outcomes will not only change my life but will definitely change the loves of those who are involved from the ground up aka "day ones." The format is contractors with the opportunities for residual and passive income. The official making for NISHW is a substantial professional accomplishment for me. We began offering CE workshops in September of 2021 and are hopeful for a full launch of our certification programs no later than Spring 2023. Sooner if all goes well. The pandemic and loss during the pandemic have deeply affected timelines, but we're incredibly proud of what we've built and what it will mean for the Sexuality field as a whole. Having an institute focused on the voices and experiences of black and brown folks is needed and will change how sexuality and the intricate parts that come along with that in communities of color. The goal is to create more qualified and equipped therapists, counselors, educators, and medical staff worldwide.

Creating a platform for us to receive quality education and supervision that will better equip us to assist in advancing sexual health in the lives of those who look like us, although a considerable accomplishment, is not what I'm most proud of. Yet, being an ally for over twenty years, not just in words but in actions, is my life's work. Being an ally is often a term that is overused and misunderstood. Recognizing Pride Month, having a gay friend, or waving a rainbow flag is NOT what allyship is about. In a world that is so critical of whom one may love, what's between their legs, and how this may differ from what's on a birth certificate from 50 years ago, the last thing we need is a closeted ally. Some say allies are not helpful. Having people who believe you should be treated differently is not enough. I agree there have been many times where I've had to have heated discussions, arguments routed in hate, discrimination and bigotry, and more to defend situations involving those highly marginalized and oppressed. I genuinely believe that being an ally, at least an ally in action, requires a level of outspokenness and refusal to be silenced for not only what you think but what many people believe are fundamental human rights for those within the LGBTQ+ community. But unfortunately, some may not want to ruffle feathers or have the hard conversations necessary to be an ally in action. This sometimes includes calling people out on their privilege and when it is showing. So therefore, they stay silent, sit around those who make discriminatory remarks, have biased conversations, or hide behind the blanket of religion to perpetuate bigotry. Not me!

I remember two instances where I have been around a group of fellow clinicians who claimed to be allies or minimally a friendly space for the LGBTQ+ community. One time, in particular, stands out that I would like to share now. I remember being on the cruise to Cuba for my first book launch. There was a specific interaction connecting with someone who was a Facebook friend. I assured her that this was a safe space for those within the community. As a member of the board, I knew this to be true. I remember introducing her to other members of this organization, fellow co-authors, and patrons on this cruise who joined us in our celebration.

There was a candid conversation that took place later that night in the dining hall. The discussion was about this person's sexual orientation and the fact that they perform cunnilingus instead of fellatio. I must have gotten up and returned to the table to this person with tears in their eyes. The level of pain and hurt that I saw in this person's body language was visibly disturbing. I remember asking what happened when I got up? They told me this was about something wrong with her because this person doesn't give head. I remember watching her argue to defend her relationship and sexuality while everyone else laughed and made a mockery of it. There were at least seven of us at this table. Most of which were licensed therapists and our psychologists who claimed to be allies or, at the very minimum, LGBTQ+ friendly. They were making a mockery at the expense of this person's sexuality. This wasn't the first test of my allyship or my beliefs, for that matter, but this one stood out to me. My response to some may have been extreme, but to me, being called out for oppressive and discriminatory comments fit the offense. I remember being so upset that this very person that I had told that this was a safe and affirming space for her was literally at the point of tears after being ridiculed and made a mockery of her sexuality. Before I knew it, I went off. Voice was raised and body language to match. I let every single one of the people around that table that we're bringing this young lady to tears about her sexuality and understand that this is entirely inappropriate for one. I didn't care if we were on a cruise. I didn't care if someone was celebrating her birthday. I also didn't care that the person was under the influence of alcohol. Mocking someone's sexuality and making the person feel like they have to get into a debate to defend what sexual acts she prefers to engage in versus those they are averse to is entirely inappropriate. I went on to tell them that I was disappointed that they called themselves allies, are supposed to be LGBTQ+ friendly, and engaged in this behavior with a colleague in the worst way.

I concluded the conversation by letting them know that I was disappointed that they had failed the organization they were there to represent today. It would not continue to happen on my watch, and I wasn't going to stand around for it. I apologized to the young lady for her experience because that was the least, I could do. I had assured her this was a safe space because I thought it was. I was wrong. The next day multiple people who were there that were authors in the book and/or observers or attendees for our cruise celebration came up to me and expressed that they had heard when it happened. They were both disappointed and saddened that this occurred in what was supposed to be a safe space. I was not ashamed of my actions from the day before. For I had showed up in a way that was affirming.

I had shown up in a way that let those around me know that no matter who you are, there was no way that I was going to allow someone to be mistreated because of their gender, sex, sexuality, or any other characteristic that was different. The rest of the cruise went smoothly, and we enjoyed Cuba and the Bahamas, but my relationship with some of those folks was never the same. And because of who I am, it could never be the same. Being an ally is about showing up when it matters. It's about having hard conversations. It's about stepping on toes and hurting feelings. It's about making sure that people know that this is not okay. You (I, People, We?) cannot use the intricate parts of someone's identity as a weapon to hurt or punish them and think that is okay.

I wish that I could say that this was the only situation in which I had to call out mental health professionals for their language in our behavior around the marginalized community that I specialize in, but it isn't.

I had another incident with a group of licensed mental health professionals for a business venture. Yes, as licensed professionals we have an ethical obligation to maintain a level of competence and awareness when it comes to client interaction and things that involve the mental health field. The conversation was around the definition of a couple. In most instances, we go with the Merriam-Webster—definition of a couple. As sexuality professionals, we understand that couples don't always look like two or people of the opposite gender or gender identity. And this could be two or more people joined together in a romantic or non-romantic way. The point of the discussion was not necessarily to find agreement and how to define a couple. It was more about having the conversation that pertained to the training we were created to ensure that we were creating something aligned with the original project's vision.

The vision is to create a very inclusive, safe, and diverse training for couples, counselors, and coaches. In addition, it would equip them to handle those seeking the help of different relationships, love styles, genders and gender identities, sexualities, kinks, and other non-traditional identifiers. Instead, what happened in this discussion was privileged that the heterosexual monogamous category showed up. However, it did so in a way that felt like erasure was taking place. Statements like "not necessary" were utilized. Verbiage about how others may feel uncomfortable with us redefining the definition of a couple. At that moment, I took a step back. I continued to listen, and then I proceeded to talk. I advised this group of female entrepreneurs, that also happened to be licensed clinical professionals, that what I am hearing is a privilege. I went on to inform them that when they are a part of the majority, they may not always see the different point of view or impact that your words, or lack thereof, may have. I expressed that their privilege was showing, and it caused me to feel that myself and others with some of my identities would feel unwelcome or excluded from this training. How we look at couples and partnerships in black and brown communities is not aligned. Then at that moment, I felt hurt, betrayed, ignored, and a lot of other feelings. However, I felt proud that I didn't sit in silence. That I didn't make the excuse of peace and not call out exclusionary behavior right when I saw it. This conversation led to heightened emotions and the potential for hurt feelings. But I never shied away from it. Instead, I addressed it head-on and confronted it in a way conducive to nurturing and courageous conversation.

The purpose of the conversation was never to sway someone to believe what I believed. I think how I think and sure as hell not to live how I live, but to recognize that being a heterosexual, monogamous, partnered, or non-partnered person comes with privilege. Those who are not heterosexual, monogamous, other gender loving, and partnered have freedom in this heteronormative world. This conversation challenges belief systems. It caused folks to look at blind spots that they may have despite saying, "I work with gay people, or I've had transgender clients before, and I didn't see a problem with it." Being open enough to see the clients or holding space for those with varied identities in business establishments is not enough. Are we able to see this person as an equal human being? Are we able to hold space for the oppression, discrimination, prejudice, and systematic attack on their basic of human rights when we can't see how our very own privilege impacts how we view the world?

This was just another example of how being an ally in action can show up. We are bombarded with biased discussions, discriminatory questions, and so much more daily in the media and social media. Our current political climate is one in which the target is on the lives, relationships, and rights of the LGBTQ+. This is an uphill battle, as the community's fundamental rights are at stake. It has led me to pursue my original career choice from fifth grade, law. The plan is to begin studying for the LSAT in 2023, pass that exam six months later, and be accepted into an HBCU Law program by 2024–2025. The types of law I plan to practice will be Civil Rights Law, Family Law, and Intellectual Property Law. With a primary focus on assisting the LGBTQ+ community. I would be a better help on the legal side of things now than on this helping one. After all, the various state governors, especially mine in Florida, trying to throw me in jail or label me as a pedophile in 2022 as a sex therapist for children, teens, and adults. My goal is to fully launch all programs at the National Institute for Sexual Health & Wellness and continue the desire to strengthen the presence and representation of black and brown sexuality professionals.

If you're genuine about inclusivity, safe, affirming spaces, and social justice for all, create and support businesses and legislation that can create effective change. This may look like the following; casting your votes during mid-term and primary elections, contacting and lobbying your state representatives, collaboration with people of color and/or getting actively involved in organizations that are BIPOC specific. It is also helpful to become involved in other major predominantly white institutions, organizations and missions that are focused on social justice and equality. After all, if you're not part of the solution, you're part of the problem.

Questions for Reflection

1. How does your current belief system differ from the one you grew up with? How might it be similar?
2. How are you actively pursuing allyship professionally or personally?
3. What are some ways that you possess privilege? Is it used to help yourself or others?
4. What is a dream or passion that you haven't followed? What's preventing you from pursuing this now?
5. How does your business plan represent inclusiveness of persons with different sexual identities?

6 Threading the Needle
Ethical Practice with Kinky Clients

Stefani Goerlich

Introduction

Since the field of Modern Psychology was introduced to the world in 19th-century Vienna, practitioners have explored the ways in which the forces of consciousness, community, and connection influence our behavior, decision making, and relationships. From Freud's analysis of the Victorian hysteric and Harlow's tactile attachment experiments, to Zimbardo's social power and authority experiments, through Watson and Rayners horrific use of sensory distress with Little Albert, researchers and clinicians have studied and sought to influence the ways in which control, authority, and sensation drive human behavior and relationships. It is no surprise then that these are the very same forces that BDSM practitioners play with in their own power exchange relationships:

Bondage and Discipline: The Exchange of Control
Dominance and Submission: The Exchange of Authority
Sadism and Masochism: The Exchange of Sensation

Today, somewhere between 2% and 8% of the population identify as kinky, or as BDSM practitioners. In the United States, this conservative 2% figure represents approximately 6.5 million people. Unfortunately, kinky people have historically faced extensive stigma from the mental health community. Kink-identified people were considered dangerously sinful in the 15th to 16th centuries (in some areas, being burned at the stake alongside witches, heretics, homosexuals, and Jews). In the 18th century, thanks to the criminal antics of the Marquis de Sade, they were often imprisoned as sexual deviants. The more "enlightened" 19th century recontextualized kinky people not as dangerous sinners, but as insane and needing institutional confinement. This remained the case throughout the 20th century, where Sadomasochism specifically was seen as a pathology to be diagnosed and eliminated. Only in very recent years has the Diagnostic and Statistical Manual's verbiage on paraphilias been rewritten to acknowledge that consensual kink is not, in and of itself, a problematic behavior. This change is

DOI: 10.4324/9781003314660-6

due in large part to the advocacy and educational efforts of mental health providers who are, themselves, kinky.

Being a Kinky Clinician

If approximately 2–8% of Americans identify as kinky, and we know there are roughly 200,000 mental health providers in the United States, back-of-the-napkin math tells us that there are (conservatively) around 4,000 kink-identified clinicians working today. These folks work in every field—from child welfare to geriatrics and include a vast spectrum of kink diversities. Some kinky clinicians enjoy solo play with the fetish object of their preference. Others are living in 24/7 power exchange relationships. Most fall somewhere in between (or on both!) points of this axis. For many, their kink identities are entirely separate and distinct from their professional work. However, there are many kink-identified providers who choose to make their knowledge and lived experience of BDSM an integral part of their clinical work. Whether they are solo practitioners or working in large provider groups, they share their expertise with the clients they serve as therapists, coaches, or healthcare providers. As with any area of special interest, the way this knowledge is embodied by the provider and shared with their clients tends to fall along a spectrum:

Kink-Curious	Kink-Informed	Kink-Aware	Kink-Affirming
Familiar with BDSM/Kink in pop culture	Has received some 101-level kink training	Seeks out ongoing learning, both academic and community	Teaches about / advocates for BDSM community
May have read fiction with BDSM themes	Reads mainstream non-fiction resources	Engages with the BDSM community outside of practice	Stays current on both academic research and community writings
May have experimented with light kink play	Comfortable discussing kink broadly with clients	Offers specific strategies to support kinky clients & relationships	Able to integrate BDSM & kink into client's treatment planning
Positive about kink but possibly carrying some myths/misconceptions	Knowledgeable enough debunk myths/misconceptions	Proactive works to dispel stigmas	Extends reach to populations marginalized within kink

Balancing self-disclosure of one's own life, relationships, and sexuality with the need to be a neutral sounding board for the client's own emotional processing is one of the most challenging aspects of being a kinky clinician. Navigating the ability to offer psychoeducation, specific suggestions (à la PLISSIT), and community resources to the kinky (or kink-curious) client while also maintaining professional boundaries can be a difficult needle to thread. This chapter provides an overview for how the kinky clinician can embody their authentic selves and offer a type of specialized client support that most other mainstream mental health providers cannot, while also maintaining appropriate professional ethics and avoiding the pitfalls of dual relationships and transference/countertransference.

Professional Ethics Overview

Whether you are a Licensed Professional Counselor, a Psychologist, a Clinical Social Worker, or a Marriage and Family Therapist, you undoubtedly have a professional code of ethics and state licensure regulations to which you are bound. The APA, NASW, ACA, and AAMFT each have language related to sexual relationships with clients.

APA: Sections 10.05, 10.06, 10.07, and 10.08 state that psychologists should not engage in sexual intimacies with current clients, relatives/significant others of current clients, or former clients. It likewise specifies that a psychologist should not act as therapist for a former sexual partner (APA, 2017). The APA does not specify what qualifies as sexual intimacy.

NASW: Section 1.09 states that "Social workers should under no circumstances engage in sexual activities, inappropriate sexual communications… or sexual contact with current clients, whether such contact is consensual or forced" (NASW, 2020). This prohibition extends to client's relatives and significant others, as well as former clients. Section 1.10 prohibits physical contact with clients, which could be construed as extending to non-sexual BDSM sensory play such as flogging.

ACA: Section A.5 prohibits sexual or romantic relationships between counselors and their current clients, their romantic partners and family members. Counselors cannot engage in a sexual or romantic relationship with a former client until five years after the termination of their professional relationship. The ACA also speaks to the prospect of sharing a BDSM/kink space with a client in Section A.6.b

Counselors consider the risks and benefits of extending current counseling relationships beyond conventional parameters…In extending these boundaries, counselors take appropriate professional precautions such as informed consent, consultation, supervision, and documentation to ensure that judgment is not impaired and no harm occurs.

(ACA, 2014)

AAMFT: Section 1.3 advises MFTs to "make every effort to avoid conditions and multiple relationships with clients that could impair professional judgment or increase the risk of exploitation" (AAMFT, 2015). Sections 1.4 and 1.5 state that sexual intimacy with current or former clients, or with known members of the client's family system is prohibited (ibid.). The AAMFT does not specify what qualifies as sexual intimacy.

These are USA-centric examples of the prohibitions (some of which are written in vague terms open to interpretation) put forth by our professional organizations. The wise clinician would see the guidance of their respective organization's ethics team, as well as legal guidance regarding the laws regulating your field's conduct within your home state or home country, before entering into kink spaces that may be shared in common with your clients.

Self-Disclosure Pros and Cons

One important factor to keep in mind when weighing the pros and cons of self-disclosure is the power differential inherent in the Client/Provider relationship. Our clients come to us because they are seeking subject matter expertise (in psychology, sexuality, etc.) that they do not themselves possess. This alone creates a power imbalance in the treatment room. This power imbalance is furthered when the provider is tasked with diagnosing the client—formally applying a label to their present state that may become a part of their medical and insurance records. Additionally, in most areas mental health providers are mandatory reporters and have the authority (even if they never use it) to intervene quite dramatically in our clients lives and autonomy. For all these reasons, providers must be aware of what they choose to share and how the client may respond to these disclosures.

It can be difficult for clients to set boundaries with their providers. Even when they feel uncomfortable with a statement or decision, the client often defers to the implied expertise of their provider and assumes that this is simply "how things work." They may worry that challenging the provider could be seen as therapeutic resistance or non-compliance. In addition, they simply may not realize that they have the right to say "I don't want to know that much about you. It makes me uncomfortable." For all of these reasons, providers must carefully weigh the value of self-disclosure against the potential negative consequences their sharing might cause. There is no one correct path—each provider must do the mental calculus of evaluating several factors: the client's needs, the therapeutic value of what they'd like to share, the size of the local BDSM/kink community, the likelihood that a client might recognize someone within the personal disclosure narrative, etc. before making the decision to disclose their own kink identities or practices. It is also important to be aware of the more overarching pros and cons that come with self-disclosure.

Pros

- Transparency around the provider's identity may prevent surprises later in the therapeutic relationship.
- The client may be relieved to not have to educate you about BDSM/kink or their relationship dynamic.
- Knowing that the provider is a BDSM/kink practitioner themselves may help establish credibility in the mind of the client.
- Provider and client can build rapport through shared understanding and commonality of lived experience.
- Knowing their provider is kinky may help challenge anti-kink stigma/biases held by the client.
- Kinky providers can offer hope to the client by modeling healthy/successful integration of BDSM/kink into their lives.
- Disclosure can be affirming for the provider, allowing them to present authentically in their clinical relationships without compartmentalizing aspects of their identities.

Cons

If the client is struggling with internalized shame around their kink identities, these may be projected onto the provider:

- Clients may bring kink identities into the treatment room in ways that undermine the therapeutic relationship (a submissive client becoming deferential to a Dominant therapist, a Dominant client pushing back on/challenging a submissive therapist, client having a strong aversion to therapist's preferred fetish).
- Disclosures may shift the relationship from therapeutic to friendly peers. Clients may want to debrief community events/gossip rather than focus on addressing their treatment goals.
- Sharing your own kink experiences may cause you (or the client) to center your own approach to BDSM, which may not work for the client. There is no one correct way to be kinky.
- When working with relationship partners, they may perceive your disclosure as alliance formation/siding with the partner who is most like yourself. (The submissive therapist may be experienced as aligning with the submissive partner at the expense of the Dominant partner's needs).
- Disclosure opens the door to additional questions, which may either shift the focus off of the client and onto the therapist, or shift the nature of the relationship from therapeutic to instructional.
- Confidentially is a one-sided commitment. The client is not obligated to protect the privacy of their provider and disclosures you make in session may be shared with others.

Community Ethics Overview

Within the Kink community, there is typically an expectation of privacy and confidentiality quite similar to that of the clinical world. There is a mutual understanding that the persons and activities we (kink affirming professionals) see at a private play party or at a public dungeon space are not to be documented or shared without the explicit consent of all involved. For most kinkspaces, this policy is explicitly outlined in their code of conduct and/or membership agreement; with camera lenses being covered with stickers or phones banned entirely. At community social meet-ups (munches/sloshes) or conferences, there is often an unspoken "if you saw me here... no you didn't" agreement among attendees that is not dissimilar to the engagement expectations between a therapist and client who happen to bump into one another at the mall. In this respect, the bonds of confidentiality between client and clinician are easy to maintain. This community norm does not exempt the provider from having conversations about informed consent, safety planning, and privacy protections with their clients prior to finding themselves in such a situation.

As more kink knowledge has entered the mainstream, many people have become familiar with the term "Safe, Sane, and Consensual" which was coined by members of the New York Gay Male S/M Activists (GMSMA) committee in the early 1980's. While popular throughout the 80's and 90's, the concept was hotly debated within the burgeoning online kink community. Gary Switch, an early critic, would coin the term RACK or "Risk Aware Consensual Kink" in 1999 as a more accurate, less subjective framework instead. RACK quickly spread and became the most common risk framework used into the present day (Nomis, 2018). The 4Cs Negotiation Model (Williams, Thomas, Prior, & Christensen, 2014), recently introduced as an update to the RACK, offers an ideal format for practitioners navigating these conversations around shared community spaces with clients:

Consent: There are many kink-identified clinicians who do not engage with their local BDSM community, either out of a desire to preserve these spaces for their clients or simply because they lack interest in doing so. A kinky clinician who is active in their local community should be transparent about this fact with the client as soon as possible—ideally as a part of their initial informed consent process at intake. There are many kinky clients who may be uncomfortable with the idea of encountering their therapist at a social event or in a play space and these clients deserve the right to opt in or out of such a possibility before the therapeutic relationship is established.

Communication: While it would naturally be inappropriate for a mental health provider to share the goings-on of their personal sexual lives and relationships, it is the clinicians' responsibility to communicate with their kink-identified clients about their participation with the public-facing BDSM community. While self-disclosure around intimate lives and behaviors (such as specific sexual practices or desires) are strongly discouraged, making sure that your clients are aware of when you will be at a BDSM community event (public or private) so that they can make an informed decision regarding whether or not to attend and can have the opportunity to create specific agreements around how an incidental encounter will be handled is vital. If you (therapists) are open about your (their) kink identity with clients, you (they) may consider publishing a monthly calendar, with any upcoming out-of-office periods, holidays, speaking engagements, and public events (kinky and non) that you (they) plan to attend. This practice-wide transparency offers your kinky clients a way to know which events they might wish to discuss with you (or opt out of) ahead of time while also normalizing participation in BDSM for your non-kinky clients as well.

Caring: Your client's needs come first. This means that if they do not want to see their clinician at an event they plan to attend, you have an ethical obligation to make other plans. This limitation can be particularly difficult for clinicians practicing in an area with a small BDSM community. Consider being vulnerable with your clients about this mutual need and collaborate to find ways to respect their privacy while also affording opportunities for engagement as well. This may take the form of agreeing to a geographic radius within which you will not attend BDSM events. It might look like trading off on scheduled events (every other monthly munch, for example) with your clients. Following your client's lead in defining what feels most comfortable for them, while still acknowledging that you are both humans with needs, lives, and relationships outside the treatment room, is a path towards modeling care for them and yourself.

Caution: There are reasons why a provider will not typically see a client who is a member of their religious community or who participates in the same softball league as they do: there are risks to sharing public space with our clients. Be mindful of the potential for dual relationship formation—especially when either you or your client holds a leadership role within a given BDSM community or organization. Outside of large metropolitan areas, BDSM communities can be quite small. Discovering that your therapist is also the host of the only munch in town, or that your new client is also a judge for the local Leather competitions you'd hoped to enter can leave folks feeling caught between connecting with local support systems and exposing themselves in a way that might not feel entirely comfortable with. Be aware of the potential for transference and countertransference to form when one or both of you has the opportunity to witness the other playing in a common BDSM space. Understand that erotic attachments can form even in the most professional of clinician-client relationships and be prepared for this to escalate if one party happens to learn that the other looks particularly great in a leather corset or has great skill wielding a paddle. Know that you and the client may bring information learned about the other outside of the treatment room into your work together and have a plan prepared ahead of time for how you will address and/or contain such knowledge when it arises in a session.

Navigating Encounters in Kinky Spaces

In a perfect world, the provider's local kink community would always be large enough to afford ample opportunities for community and play without ever worrying about crossing paths with a client. The reality for many (if not most) however, is that outside of large metropolitan areas, the BDSM scene tends to be small. Everyone knows everyone else and there may only be a handful of events each year for folks to attend. In these settings, it becomes far more likely that the kink-identified provider and their client will bump into each other at some point. Many kinky providers reduce this possibility by choosing not to engage with the BDSM community in their local area. They skip the munches and play parties, and choose to leave these to be the exclusive domain of their clients. This is the most surefire way to avoid uncomfortable encounters in kinky spaces. Other kinky providers set the boundary differently—they will attend social events that do not involve play, such as educational events or social meet-ups (the aforementioned munch) but avoid dungeon spaces or play parties. Still others decide that living authentically as a kinky clinician means embodying their full selves—even if this might mean crossing paths with a client while in a state of undress or encountering them during a scene.

The standard practice here is the same as when we encounter a client anywhere else: we do not acknowledge, greet, or approach them. Depending upon the event, the choice a provider makes from there may vary. At a large social gathering or educational event, it may be possible to stay in the same room, buffered by the crowd, and simply avoid interaction. In more intimate settings, however, a choice must be made. Many providers will choose to leave an event once they've become aware of a client's presence. This allows them to preserve the therapeutic distance necessary for an effective working relationship while also not asking the client to give up or lose out on an enjoyable social event. Even here, this must be handled with tact. If a client walks into the room and you immediately stand and start gathering your things, that can raise questions as well. Making your exit quietly and unobtrusively, leaving enough time between the client's arrival and your departure that you don't draw attention to the two, is key here.

The situation becomes a little trickier when a therapist encounters a client in a dungeon space or at a play party. The nature of such settings is usually rather dark, and depending upon the evening's activities (say, if blindfolds are involved) one or both you may not immediately see one another. Some providers will simply move to another room and take pains to avoid being in physical proximity to their clients for the duration of the evening. Others will take the client's presence as their cue to exit. The latter is the safest solution, from a licensure and liability perspective.

There can arise rare instances where a provider takes all necessary steps to preserve their client's agency and their own privacy, and still encounter complicated situations. Perhaps you decide on a personal policy of avoiding your local BDSM community and only engaging with kinksters in the next large city. Your partners who do not share this same restriction may still encounter people who are your clients. At the most extreme, there have been instances where a provider has realized that their partner engaged in a pick-up scene with a client at a party they took pains to avoid themselves. Obviously, it is impossible to disclose to your partner your relationship to the client, however it is still necessary to address this complicated situation. Often, the solution is to refer the client out. However, this often feels unfair. After all, the client did nothing to warrant the loss of a beneficial therapeutic relationship! In these scenarios, often the only person aware of the ethical concern is the provider themselves. This is why, when a local BDSM community is particularly small, many providers choose to avoid it entirely. The best way to prevent ethical conflicts is to simply not insert oneself into situations that could cause them to arise.

Liability Concerns

As discussed, most of the professional codes of ethics are vague about what they call sexual intimacy. It is incredibly important, therefore, to seek the guidance of both your state licensing board and your professional liability insurance provider to determine what is considered ethical practice if you plan on being fully out as a kinky clinician. Many sexual harassment laws are written to include verbal harassment or unwanted sexual speech, and if your client is uncomfortable with personal disclosure in session, you may inadvertently find yourself at the receiving end of an ethics complaint. This becomes even more crucial when we consider somatic practice and more hands-on education that often occurs under the auspices of coaching. If you are a licensed mental health provider, be very clear about what behaviors (from verbal disclosures to attending kink events where clients are to marketing yourself as a "kink coach") are protected and which open you up to liability concerns. Ethics complaints, even those that do not result in formal disciplinary action, are reflected on your license in many states and may result in an increase in your insurance premiums or even a loss of coverage entirely. The single safest way to protect your practice and your license is to avoid personal disclosures about your BDSM practices and direct engagement with your local kink community. That said, this is an unacceptable sacrifice for many providers, who deserve to have the same level of community connection and support that our clients do. If you fall into this category, approach your public facing kink from a RACK (Risk-Aware Consensual Kink) perspective and do the necessary research to prevent ethical issues further down the road.

Setting Boundaries Outside of the Practice Space

Many mental health providers do not limit their practice to just direct client contact. They are also clinical supervisors, adjunct faculty, researchers, conference speakers, guest lecturers, media voices, authors, and more. When you are public-facing as a kinky clinician, or even a kink-affirming clinician, it naturally evokes questions from others about what drew you to this particular area of specialty. If you are comfortable being outspoken about your personal kink identities, this can be a wonderful time to challenge cultural biases and misconceptions about kinky people. However, the vast majority of kinksters are not living their lives as open books. In the same way that we do not discuss our sexual habits with our children or parents; we do not ask the stranger in the grocery line how their intimate relationships are structured. There is nothing unprofessional or inappropriate about setting strong boundaries around what you are willing to share about your life with others—even others who know you work with the BDSM community.

Dr. Ruth Westheimer is most famous as one of the first "celebrity" sexologists. Over the course of her career, she had a call-in radio show that ran for a decade (at the height of the AIDS crisis), a television show which drew two million viewers per week, hosted several cable TV shows and wrote over 30 books. Dr. Ruth talked about everything from homosexuality to herpes, from pedophilia to premature ejaculation. For over 50 years she has talked about any and every kind of sex, but one—the kind she had with her own partner. Dr. Ruth is a role model of how to embody shame-free, sex positive, public advocacy without needing to violate one's own boundaries to do so. When you are asked questions about your own personal life or kink identity, you may have different boundaries than hers. However, it behooves the ethical provider to be judicious and discerning not only in what we share, but with who. Before answering questions about your own sexual practices or relationships, consider exploring the intent behind the question a bit first. Try using one of the following responses, before defaulting to a personal disclosure:

- "That's an interesting question. What brings it up?"
- "I wonder why you're curious about my private life."
- "No, I won't answer that. A better question might be…"
- "How would you respond if someone asked you about your intimate life?"
- "I'd rather not personalize this conversation. What interests me most about the topic is…"

- "My peers and I often debate how much of our personal lives to share with others. Where do you think that line should be?"
- "I'm wondering how knowing that would be helpful to you right now?"
- "I'm asked that question a lot, and it always makes me feel..."

Being a sexual health professional does not obligate you to use your own life and relationships as object lessons. Redirecting questions that feel intrusive, or simply unnecessary, away from yourself and back towards the general knowledge we hope to impart as sexuality advocates is one of the most important skills the provider can develop—and our ability to do so, politely and cheerfully, empowers our clients to do the same in their own lives and relationships.

Marketing yourself as a Kink-Affirming Practitioner

Being kinky yourself is not sufficient to market yourself as a kink-affirming practitioner. As with any other therapeutic modality, clinicians are obligated to undertake the necessary learning and skill-building required to ethically make a claim to practice. Before marketing yourself as kink-affirming, ask yourself the following questions:

- Am I familiar with the Clinical Practice Guidelines for Working with People with Kink Interests?
- Do I keep apprised of the latest research on kink sexuality, relationships, and mental health?
- Do I have a strong background in Sexual Health knowledge, including physiological, medical, gender diversity, reproductive justice issues, STI prevention, etc.?
- Do I have training in Relationship or partnership counseling, such as The Gottman Method, Relational Life Therapy, Imago, or Emotionally Focused Therapy?
- Do I have training in Kink-Specific Mental Health knowledge? (*The Alternative Sexual Health Alliance/TASHRA, Sexual Health Alliance/SHA, and The Buehler Institute, among others, offer a variety of trainings on this subject.*)
- Have I learned from the lived experience of kinksters, by listening to podcasts, reading community-published books, attending BDSM conferences, etc.?
- Do I have a thorough foundation in the psycho-social history of BDSM, how kinky people have been treated (legally, spiritually, and socially) over the last 250 years?

- Am I aware of the variety of BDSM/kink *subcultures*, their nuances, commonalities, and distinctions? (See chart below for a non-exhaustive list of kink subcommunities.)
- Do I understand the ways in which Old Guard Leather and the early LGBTQI+ communities overlapped, cross-pollinated, and supported one another? Can I describe the role that kinky people played in the Pride and civil rights movements?
- Is my practice grounded in the principles of Intimate Justice and Pleasure Equity?

Adult Baby/ Diaper Lovers (ABDL)	Fetishistic role play wherein one partner assumes the persona of an infant/toddler, including diaper wearing/usage, bottle/ breastfeeding, etc. while the other takes on the role of nurturing caregiver.
Caregiver/Little	Power exchange dynamic wherein the Dominant partner takes on a more gentle/supportive authority role (often called Mommy/Daddy Dom) encouraging their submissive partner to assume a more childlike or innocent demeanor, often including regressive age play.
Domestic Discipline/50s Household	Authority exchange relationship characterized by a highly patriarchal, typically (but not exclusively) heteronormative "traditional" nuclear family. Often includes fetishization of mid-century aesthetics and styles. This dynamic can also be found within traditionalist ("Trad") Evangelical relationships disconnected from the broader kink community.
FinDom	Power exchange relationships wherein the submissive person ("Pay Pig") cedes financial authority and control of their personal accounts, including ATM codes and sensitive money management data, to a Dominant who humiliates them by spending or taking their money.
Gorean	A form of M/s based on the fantasy Gor Novels, written by John Norman. These works have heavily influenced BDSM culture, however many consider them to be misogynistic and homophobic today. Gorean households are male dominated and emphasize humiliation, service, and objectification of submissives referred to as kaijiras.
Master/Slave	A style of consensual authority and control-based power exchange wherein the submissive partner considers themselves to be the wholly owned property of their Dominant Master. These relationships often involve some form of 24/7 submission, as well as an agreement that the submissive partner is voluntarily giving up their right to say no to their Dominant. The term Master/slave is beginning to fall out of favor in the US due to an increased sensitivity to the use of language in relation to the nation's history of forced enslavement, however M/s is still commonly used within much of the global BDSM community.

(Continued)

Pet/Pony Play	Fetishistic power exchange dynamic wherein the submissive role plays as an animal (puppy, kitten, pony, pig, etc.) and the Dominant acts as their trainer/handler or owner. Often includes elements of play, physical activity, and the use of masks or other wearables designed to dehumanize the submissive and reinforce their animal state.
Primal/Prey	A form of non-structured power exchange, emphasizing the emotional experience and physicality of hunting, chasing, and capturing. These relationships typically eschew honorifics and rituals/protocol and often allow for more egalitarian sensory play (biting, wrestling, etc.) between partners.
Riggers/Rope Players	Term used for individuals who enjoy rope play: shibari, suspension, restraint using rope, etc. Considered an exchange of control, rope play may or may not include other power exchange elements such as authority or sensation exchange. Note: persons who enjoy being tied in ropes are sometime called "rope bunnies." Many consider this term to be demeaning. Practitioners should avoid its use.
Technosexuals	Individuals who fetishize elements of technology as an aspect of their kink play or who experience sexual desire for tech-based partners such as robots, holograms, or AI devices.

If you choose to market yourself as a kink-friendly or kink-affirming provider, it is possible to list yourself as such on platforms such as TherapyDen and PsychologyToday. The National Coalition for Sexual Freedom also maintains a Kink Affirming Providers directory that lists professions raging from mental health providers to CPAs and everything in between. Putting language on your website such as "my practice is informed by the Clinical Guidelines for Working with People with Kink Interests" can be very reassuring to potential clients; as can the inclusion of symbols such as the BDSM triskelion or the Leather Pride flag. Another great way to reach potential kinky clients is to advertise at local kink events or regional conferences. Even if you've made a decision not to attend yourself, reaching out to the organizers and inquiring about sponsorship opportunities can put your name and practice on the minds of dozens, if not hundreds, of potential new clients. Even when your client panel is full, sponsoring local community events is a wonderful way to build your brand and your reputation as a kinky clinician.

Somatic Work and Coaching with Kinky Clients

There are some mental health professionals and sexuality educators who choose to engage in more somatic forms of work with their clients. This can take the form of surrogate partnerships, hands-on kink education, or BDSM coaching. If you are professionally licensed, be mindful of the limitations of your liability protections when it comes to somatic work and coaching practices. Often, these services are perceived by the client to be similar enough to kink-affirming therapy to be misconstrued as a form of treatment. If you choose to engage in somatic work or coaching, the best practice would be to keep this quite separate and distinct from your work as a clinician. Some would argue that one should avoid these practices entirely, unless your therapeutic practice is entirely disconnected from your somatic or coaching work. For example, a kink-affirming Certified Sex Therapist who also offers hands-on BDSM coaching to clients in the local dungeon space is far more likely to blur ethical boundaries than a Licensed Professional Counselor who works as a substance use treatment counselor from 9–5 and then does the same.

It is our responsibility as professionals to protect our clients from harm. Harm can come in many forms, from inadvertent outing as a client or a kinkster, to the emotional pain of erotic transference, to the potential for sexual exploitation or abuse. Setting and maintaining clear boundaries around our personal and professional sexualities and sexual expression is the key to reducing the risk of harm to our clients and ourselves. Carefully consider your personal needs, professional goals, ethical standards, and tolerance for risk before engaging in direct physical interactions (i.e., somatic touch or a shibari workshop) with the clients who you treat.

Conclusion

The world has changed dramatically for kinky people over the last 25 years. The DSM now clearly states that consensual kink is not enough to warrant a paraphilia diagnosis. More and better BDSM cultural competency education is available to mental health practitioners across the spectrum. Power exchange relationships and sensory play have entered the popular mainstream in ways that no longer portray kinksters as either a serial killer or seductress. And more and more kink-identified clinicians are bringing their enthusiasm for kink and personal experiences with BDSM positivity into the treatment room. These are all positive changes and we should continue to encourage more and greater open dialogue around sexuality and relationship diversity. Doing so ethically requires more reflection and risk awareness for kinky clinicians, but the benefits (to both clients and community) are well worth it.

Questions for Reflection

1. Why might some sexuality professionals be resistant to having more kink aware and affirming practices?
2. What do you think the general public needs to know about kink communities in order to have more expansive dialogue?

3. In your opinion, should kink affirming practice be taught in graduate and postgraduate programs or should it be considered an outside specialty?
4. What are some of the challenges and advantages for kink professionals to self-disclose?
5. What is your theoretical perspective and how does it include discussions about fantasy, desire, and kink in your clinical practice?

References

AAMFT. (2015). *Code of Ethics*. Retrieved from American Association for Marriage and Family Therapy: https://aamft.org/Legal_Ethics/Code_of_Ethics.aspx

ACA. (2014). *2014 ACA Code of Ethics*. Retrieved from American Counseling Association: chrome-extension://efaidnbmnnnibpcajpcglclefindmkaj/https://www.counseling.org/resources/aca-code-of-ethics.pdf

APA. (2017). *Ethical Principles of Psychologists and Code of Conduct*. Retrieved from American Psychological Association: https://www.apa.org/ethics/code?item=13#1005

NASW. (2020). *Code of Ethics*. Retrieved from National Association of Social Workers: https://www.socialworkers.org/About/Ethics/Code-of-Ethics/Code-of-Ethics-English/Social-Workers-Ethical-Responsibilities-to-Clients

Nomis, A. O. (2018). *The History of SSC (Safe Sane Consensual) vs RACK (Risk-Aware Consensual Kink)*. Retrieved from History of the Dominatrix: https://historyofthedominatrix.com/blogs/blog/the-history-bdsm-consent-ssc-vs-rack

Williams, D., Thomas, J. N., Prior, E. E., & Christensen, M. C. (2014). From "SSC" and "RACK" to the "4Cs": Introducing a new Framework for Negotiating BDSM Participation. *Electronic Journal of Human Sexuality*, *Volume 17*, www.ejhs.org/volume17/BDSM.html.

7 Survivor to CEO
Activation in Practice

Mary May

Introduction

Leadership is a natural assignment. It comes with a special skill set for your personal and professional interests. In the scope of your roles with each new experience, you gain insight that connects you to seeking higher responsibility. Navigating how one reaches each level in their career coincides with lived experiences. Such experiences have shaped our views, perspectives, esteem, and confidence. In light of growing through each moment, the residue of surviving often is tucked and hidden once you get through it. Acknowledging this space of survival requires clarity and supported direction. If this direction is not established, you can become stagnant and feel frustrated or stuck.

Leadership being your assigned designation requires you to set the logistics with clear goals and intentions. The long-term goals challenge you to confront your current skill set and strive for the desired level and role in your professional career with opportunities. Developing a Leadership Blue Print offers you the opportunity to acquaint yourself with the step-by-step process that will guide you toward the success of your vision. In the scope of development, your position is best served by setting the coordinates of your professional GPS. In the navigation of survival to CEO there is a specialized GPS formula that breaks down the acronym into three instrumental parts 1) **Goals**—Gain clarity on your vision to gain access to where you are leveling up toward 2) **Plan/Positioning**—Once you have identified the goals you can make a clear path of your step by step process, and 3) **Strategy**—Building capacity, skill, and grit to navigate what your call to leading at a higher level requires and being able to sustain.

In this chapter, you will interrogate how your values, beliefs, and skills impact your capacity to excel. When we interrogate and/or confront areas of growth that have been intertwined with what we are surviving, conflict develops. It is generally a strong attempt to compartmentalize undesirable moments and experiences, not realizing how they shape our capacity as leaders. This is the very thing that the leadership GPS navigation will guide you through to become the CEO of your life.

DOI: 10.4324/9781003314660-7

Leaders generally have routines and patterns that propel them with a high level of motivation. Therefore, encouraging your ability to grow and seek new opportunities is imperative. It can be layered with some experiences that have conditioned your perspective to develop fear. Such fear is the thought process that may allow what you have survived, via experiences, to have unresolved residue. This prevents your success while keeping you silent and feeling unheard. Consequently, the value of survival is connected to your leadership intentions as the two coincide. Survival is defined as the act of surviving; continuing or lingering after some event.

The ability to recenter and remain focused on your development as a leader is important. This is because events that you may be surviving and growing through can detour your navigation and cause delays. We will dig deeper into how you may have encountered some roadblocks and the challenges connected to how you will be able to level up with professional opportunities. It can be complicated and simple all in the same breath. At times we have to reassess and reset our bandwidth with an effective strategy that enables us to break all glass ceilings that are in our way.

Experiencing detour after detour can cause one to doubt their ability to continue the leadership path. This is where it serves you to dig in and confront your bandwidth which can stretch your values, beliefs, skills, and challenges. Being able to push and lead forward will help you recognize that each moment and experience is shaping your skillset to confidently sustain the CEO position of your personal and professional life.

In the absence of having the clarity of infusing the GPS, you will be conditioned to be stuck and repeat the steps and patterns that have always detoured your journey. Removing the blinders takes perspective and activates an honest inventory of what undesirable experiences continuously distract you on your path. This shift will allow you to interrogate where and why you are stuck. Furthermore, being able to decrease the projection and blame on external forces such as relationships, family/partners, missed opportunities, promotion, etc., will help you pursue your leadership journey authentically.

Let's get ready to peel back the layers and position ourselves for the most beneficial solution in leadership. Recalling the role and purpose of infusing the **G.P.S.** (Goals. Positioning/Planning. Strategy) that will lead us toward being unapologetically successful.

When you don't know where you're going you begin by establishing goals or destinations. Just like when we are driving, you may initially be unclear of your direction and sometimes even the purpose of your journey. Navigation is needed to support our clarity and inner standing of what is needed to land opportunities of value that we deserve and desire. When we lock into the coordinates of the *G.P.S. Leadership Blue Print* and follow the flow with consistency, positive outcomes arise.

When you consider what the framework and formula of the GPS opens up it reveals

- **Not only** the ability to identify **GOALS**
- **Not only** the ability to identify the **PLAN**
- **Not only** the ability to identify the **STRATEGY**

It also identifies the *BLIND SPOTS* and *BARRIERS* that are keeping you from what it is that you want and provides you the side-by-side support of what is needed. Being able to be honest to work through, honor, give space and/or voice, and awareness of survival narrative because you are going to value the commitment that you make to your leadership journey.

Setting the Stage

Let's set the stage and backdrop to the layers we will scale back to launch forward. Leveling up and securing opportunities that offer you the opportunity to balance out your career and life overall enables progress. The intersection of your career and your lived experiences from survival can lean in from various places in life. This can be from a previous performance review/appraisal, critiques about your ideas, the act of overthinking, and more. Engaging and leveling up to CEO status and leadership in your life can be very complicated and overwhelming.

All of the development as a leader can be triggered by a degree of what one has encountered and is currently surviving. The experiences can at times create a trauma response that opens the survival part of our mind that invites us to compartmentalize by tucking it away. The conflicts in life that we have encountered in our lives leave untamed and unresolved energy as residue over time. As a professional, you want to believe that your professional growth is not consumed with your reaction and exposure to undesirable experiences. Consequently, we have survived many things like being passed over for promotion and salary challenges. But we have also survived other lived experiences that have an impact and influence on how we lead forward. Some of these experiences can be the transition or loss of a job, layoff, relationships, home, children, finances, fire, homelessness, divorce, abandonment, and even possible sexual violation or abuse.

These losses can overlap and even mirror interactions that will arise in your leadership interactions. This would appear by you having a different value set for your skill set and bandwidth in the workplace than your executive team views. This can become disruptive within your next-level goals as the continual denial, ignoring, and not being seen can trigger parallels to earlier experiences in your familial relationships and other adult interactions. Unintentionally, you default to the reaction of resentment and downgrade the thought process of you not being deserving of something at a higher level. If you as a leader have not become aware of this trigger and responsive behavioral pattern that you engage in over time, your goals will be activated and have a recurring roadblock or stopping point.

It can feel and appear as though you are not being seen, experiencing the respect deserved, and not receiving the financial gains of being well paid with a promotion. The infusion of the deep dive strategy of infusing the *G.P.S. Leadership Blue Print* will allow you to connect the intersectional moments and begin to unlearn prohibitive patterns so that you can excel.

This exchange in your communication with executive leaders and your colleagues develops the comparison and limits related to breaking the glass ceiling. In life, we need to pull the curtain of our dual realities back before the awareness and conceptual mind dump to learn the overlapping themes and concepts. The concept of pulling the curtain back is taking a look at hidden gems and experiences that inform your mindset and what you take action on. There is residue everywhere and because you have gotten to the management team and can envision your ability to be on the CEO platform, you can believe that previous challenges do not matter.

Surprisingly it has everything to do with each other. Your insight and ability to activate the process of moving forward is masked by other experiences where you are paused sitting at the red light in traffic, while everyone and everything else around you is growing forward in their best lane of genius possible. Hence, this creates the feeling that you have been passed over and overlooked for an opportunity. You possibly develop this narrative of incompatibility with leveling up in your leadership. Life experiences teach us when to lean forward and when to pause. Unfortunately, if we have survived some challenges, we avoid them due to comfort and fear.

Pulling back the curtain is synonymous with fall engagement and honest personal inventory to build your personalized *Leadership Blue Print*. Discovering the impact also aligns you with the influence of all parts of you, as the human first and leader second, is the very instrumental step to activating how you will develop the best strategy to get unstuck from survival mode and activate the higher version of yourself. One of the best perspectives of securing this is to do the personal and honest inventory that comes with pulling the curtain back but not getting stuck there. This takes strategy, intervention, and side-by-side support.

Confrontation is not a weakness or a challenge, it is a privilege and gift to trust your ability to create the best version of yourself. As a leader, the word "confrontation" is understood as being challenging versus a learning platform that is open to the exchange of ideas while developing your inner standing of creating life on your terms. It is the respect that you are due, with or without the credentials already secured. However, the game changer knows how you may have positioned yourself in the past and whether it was favorable for your intention to lead in this current season of life.

Again, as we look to grow forward in your leadership, improve your awareness of what you have compartmentalized from the undesirable experiences and reset the perspective on how you will integrate your growth and transition into your influence/power. This beneficial shift that can be significant in our growth is the ability to improve your awareness and be open to reset your navigation as you learn each trigger and roadblock in your plan.

It's time to NEXT LEVEL your career

Securing your promotion in a non-compartmentalized thought framework that informs you on how to navigate at your ambition level and higher. When you have done the emotional work that informs you to pause, start, activate, and sometimes pause again, this is when the interrogation of the internal dialog informs our external dialog. This takes place with the role of a delayed opportunity. Additionally, clarity is gained on what we may have allowed to intimidate and inform the internal dialog that has you doing things differently.

We are not always invisible—we become invisible by triggered inner dialog that intimidates us and our value of leading in our expertise effectively. In the navigation of the survival narratives, you are challenged with the daily divorce of self which holds all the experiences and ideas on autopilot that discourage you. Your leadership is on reset when this has been triggered, and in absence of a tool kit of confidence and conviction. you are in the right place to become silenced. As you come closer to walking in your authority with confidence daily, your routine is getting you closer to the prize of being a CEO.

Most likely, you have been very close to this space several times in your career. In some cases, you have been able to excel and in some, and in others you encounter blind spots and roadblocks. Be aware that the ripples in the journey or matrix are the simple test of your grit and fortitude to understand that the next leveling requires you to manage your emotions and process potential disappointment. The external challenges will encourage you to simply throw in the towel and be sufficient at the level you are currently living. The consequence of this is that this is not in alignment with your assignment in the scope of work that is your footprint in leadership.

You may have heard the mantra that the process is the real prize. It is the activating of doing what it takes to understand that inner dialog and the inner standing of your value as a leader. You then understand that what you have to offer is not that complicated. All things perceived as difficult are a question of whether you have done the work necessary.

Perhaps you have become comfortable with the experience of not obtaining the opportunity that you have sought. The recurrence of this has your internal dialog attempting to shift your focus toward being complacent. Depending on the residue from what you have survived, it is very closely reminiscent of how you are reacting and responding in this situation. Where is your inventory checkpoint so that you can reflect and reset, knowing that a shift is necessary to grow from being uncomfortable?

What becomes instrumental in how you position yourself has shifted your work ethic along with your commitment. The question to ask yourself is are you limiting yourself by the location of this opportunity and creating your glass ceiling? The limiting beliefs challenge our continued work ethic when we feel that we have been overlooked, invisible, and requests ignored. The impact of positioning yourself and working the plan of your G.P.S. has prepared you for this very moment while embracing your ability to succeed. When you get to this point of knowing what your process will be, your confidence begins to secure each step with the confidence and esteem that you have not experienced before. You are more than deserving and capable to be in the C-Suite version of how you envision the work-life balance with harmony.

Engaging and living in the space unapologetically causes you to shift your value of how you experience this growth of leading forward. Your goals are clear. You are positioned and walking in the plan set for you. You have been receptive to the strategy where you are routinely now cleaning up that residue that has been triggering you and keeping you stuck.

Now that you are unlocked and loaded in your influence and understanding the internal dialog that has shifted, you have a new perspective of what motivates you and your WHY.

Let's take a quick moment that will guide you in being clear about what you are allowed to experience. As a leader, you are the activator of your automatic messaging to inform your brain to unlearn the limiting values and beliefs that have driven you before now. As the driver of your success, recognize all of the overlapping intersections that drive us and allow you to activate the next version of your leading.

Then ask yourself and put in your own words:

What has been in your way?
What are the barriers that restrict your leadership role?
Have you considered that your next opportunity in leveling up may be at a different company?
What is your rationale for how you engage with others and how may that motivate the actions you activate?
What makes this the best fit for you? And the most important thing, what is your WHY?
What are two ways that you have felt overlooked, invisible, and passed over?

As you engage in this shift an honest inventory of your perspective and values change. It is important to routinely refresh the value meter of your skill set and personal values. This allows you to always be in tune to have clear insight that guides your decisions in every leading role that you engage in. Let's look at the value of a bottle of water.

The story about the value of the bottle of water is a good perspective on how worth and your value to an environment can matter.

A bottle of water in the supermarket is worth 50 cents, the same bottle of water in a bar is worth approximately $2. In a good restaurant or hotel, it can be worth up to $3 and at an airport or in another place of business it can be up to $5.

The bottle is the same, and the brand, too, can be the same. The only thing that changes is the place and positioning.

When you feel zero, you're worthless (least valuable), when everyone around you may limit interactions with you, you should change places, don't stay there. This is where the navigation plan encourages you to surround yourself with leaders at your ambition level and higher. Where their vibrations can recognize and not stifle your opportunity with limits that are not mirroring your intention and skill set. You activate where your potential will rise and excel. You are also motivated to lead and share from a positive framework utilizing your strengths. These spaces automatically empower your voice, mindset, and bandwidth that bring you to the desired conversations about elevated projects and promotions that will serve as growth for you.

Sometimes the location is everything. The destination of a leader is ever-evolving and does not have to be locked and loaded where you have been, but have a designation where you are empowered while leveling up. Be open to the time to change location and position to create the work-life balance within the career you deserve.

Have the courage to change your circle and go to a place where they give you the courage you deserve, and consider **YOU**, who you are and what you have to offer to the overall goal. Surround yourself with people who appreciate your worth and what you contribute to the conversation. Are you clear on what you have to offer and how you can reposition the statement of your leadership skills for managing how you would develop the life that you deserve to grow from on your terms?

Keep in mind that as you continue to go through this experience, each place has a different value for the same bottle of water as described above. When you feel like you are worth nothing and your contribution is not valued, it is time to *RESET* and get *SNATCHED*. Leveling up to a **S.N.A.T.C.H.E.D.** version of leadership means that you have learned how to navigate from both sides of leadership with **S**trategic **N**etworking and **A**lliances yield **T**ransformative **C**ollaborations that **H**elp **E**nergize **D**evelopment.

Do you need your team, manager, etc., to celebrate what you contribute to their continued growth? It is time to change the places and not stay at a standstill where you are being belittled and your wings clipped so that you can excel with all of the potentials that you bring to leadership.

The glass ceiling is a loaded narrative that many examples and experiences can be offered and provided. When you think of the glass ceiling, it is important to think about being limited, smothered, and challenged to breathe and create. It may also be manifested via micro/macro-aggressions that we encounter on a daily swivel in the workplace. As an elevating leader, your growth is tempered by experiences that manifest triggers that can harm your ability to level up. How you infuse them in your navigation of leadership, with communication and resolving, is another instrumental game changer that positions you for the CEO lifestyle that you seek.

In various levels of leadership there are many ways that you can impact and influence change with yourself first and with the team members that work with you. You may already have a seat at the table but not the positioning that will allow your vision, purpose and value to the conversation to lead due to differences and perspective taking from other members at the same said table.

One of the factors behind goal setting and the distractions away from your commitment is informed from various characteristics that exist in our work culture. The boundaries, ethics and varying degrees of cultural acceptance and/or denial in the work space causes conflict of your performance and capability in leadership. You may have applied to various opportunities and are unclear on what the blind spots that you are unaware of and why the roadblock exists. The tricky thing is that it can have something to do with your presentation but it can also have something to do with understanding the culture of your team.

There are social pressures that we ignore that exist as micro/macro aggressions that impact how we interact with executive leadership. The influence of power dynamics, gender biases, the need for validation, and other emotional reactions also play a role. When you are leaving the meeting that has occurred and your suggestions and feedback have been dismissed, ignored, and sometimes shared by other team members and accepted—causes emotional injury in the workplace. When you take on the defensive role, it may not be communicated with the value that you bring but all emotion. The reasons behind why validation and your voice being heard is fueled from previous contact here at work but also in your personal lives. How you engage (proactive/dwelling) can often be viewed by executive leadership that you may not be able to handle the swift decision making and high-level conversations.

Your mind and body are attempting to balance the fight or flight response on a daily basis. There are coping skills that you have created to manage the stress that is created in your daily interactions as you attempt to recover from the recurring experiences. The continual stress our body feels that it has to protect us and that we have to remap how we react versus creating thoughtfulness in managing and making effective decisions.

In the list above, we are attempting to regulate these moments in the workplace that create stress just as it has when we were in survival mode in other areas of our lives. Symptoms of headaches, stomach pain, irritability, and a high level of incapacity make us believe that we are not prepared to level up in our career. The body takes about 90 minutes after each reaction to the body and mind, thinking that it has to protect us with thoughts being rehearsed over and over again. You will begin to understand what you have survived, how it is playing a part in your daily leadership roles, and how it paralyzes your ability to level up effectively. When is it okay to let your guard down? Let's create thoughtful space to understand that the unknown outcomes that we cannot control are not scary but beneficial.

Survival and GRIT

Let's get **S.N.A.T.C.H.E.D.** You have your credentials, and certificates and have been dedicated to your career for some time. You are exhausted with the efforts in securing your next level and promotion. In some cases, you have been permitted to play in the game of interim position here and there but not securing the official WIN.

You have tasted the balance of life with vacations, and hanging with friends and family but that gets snatched every time you have a NEW project, contract, or life just seems to happen. The download from lived experiences and even from growing up is that we put our ALL into what we are working on and we will receive our reward. However, it seems like your work is being overlooked, ignored, stolen, or that you are downright invisible.

Now, look—there comes a time when you have to confront and do something uncomfortable to get that level-up experience that will reset your life and experience that will balance your decisions out effectively. At this point, you have made several investments in your life but there is something unresolved and untamed that is impacting your ability to have success in the conference room and translate into your leadership. How you view what you have accomplished is success in the short-term experience. As a leader you are best served in your awareness of your value. Your value is the strong confidence that sustains your leadership. Your productivity and performance strategy did not just create itself. It has been a part of who you are at the core but, at the same time, you need to pause to look at what you have survived in your lifetime.

At this point in your career in leadership, you have navigated several situations as you have become accomplished. You have also been able to work and grow through the many social constructs that are put in the path to detour your focus and challenge the capability of doing the work. The workplace has expectations that vary from one leader to the next and at times how they define things like "professionalism" for various isms.

In light of maintaining your GRIT and stick to its nature, the construct of professionalism is ever evolving and is where the compromise of your skill does not meet workplace politics. How you speak, dress, style your hair, and respond is oftentimes highly criticized. The code switching from how you may engage socially to meet the ever-changing standard in the workplace can be exhausting. Not to mention the standard of dress that is put in place to constrict what is not understood from some of the cultural forms of expression that a leader may have. This interaction can also create roadblocks and perception is everything. At the end of the day, are you aware of what this professional exchange is triggering in you? As well as what has it to do with your performance? The ability to sustain your leadership, and not be distracted by what triggers you, takes a level of work that is also gained with infusing what is learned in the *G.P.S. Leadership Blue Print*.

We have taken a brief look at the construct and challenges of working to fit in with the construct of professionalism. However, there are many other emotional infractions that happen in leadership and in your life that can cause conflict with your ability to level up. The vicarious reaction and/or experience with personal and professional life cannot effectively be compartmentalized. You are encouraged to take a personal and honest inventory with your journey that has shaped how you lead today.

When you have experienced hardship that either you have ignored or worked through in silence, it can result in residue that impacts your leadership. Some of the experiences can be a result of insecurity with housing, food, and finances, divorce as a child and/or in your adult relationships, seasons with anxiety, abandonment, sexual assault, and depression. This shift can alter your perspective and productivity. While your leadership is impacted, there are also some strengths that have been gained from these least desired experiences. If you have ignored the presence of how they impacted how you navigate life, it is possible to show up at the most inopportune time. Generally, it is when you are seeking promotion and positioning yourself to level up with all of your experience and credentials.

Due to the survival narrative that you have developed over time, you may think that it is not necessary to consider the impact. Consequently, there are adverse effects that, even if years have passed, can impact how you excel in the conference room and high-level engagement in your journey to CEO. Your ability to communicate, establish trust, and mutual boundaries that are sufficient in the professional role is key. The ability to shift from the performance narrative from a distant and cold position will develop the personal character that sustains your desired role in leadership. The infusion and support that is provided in the *G.P.S. Leadership Blue Print* is your personalized script of learning how to navigate with value. This will ultimately give you the space and authority to not get stuck and distracted but to continue your focus and intention leading forward without the roadblock.

Self-care is a RESET beyond getting a massage, nails, and hair done. Accountability is the RESET of changed behavior and a SHIFT in your codependency to the survival voice that paralyzes you. It's time to create the strategy and pull the curtain back so that you can step to the center of the stage with conviction, value, and belief that you DESERVE to EXCEL. When you remember and confidently believe you are who you say you are, the competition is over and you don't have to prove it to others

The IDEA of Perfection

Anxiety is on overload. We are empowered by avoidance. Being Busy. Procrastination delays being authentic in our super energy. (Perfection is an anxiety playground). However, in this download of the life, we have lived and experienced. We have also been exposed to conflicting with our lower-valued thoughts and actions. We have a viewpoint of where they have started but it is time to burn the connection that we have to them so that we can effectively elevate and level up.

Let's take a moment to unlock the *RED LIGHT MAGIC*. You have a new idea in your life as a leader or personal development. You share with someone you trust and they do not agree with this or share some contrary benefits. Because you value their voice and opinion and it does not align with you—you are paused, rethinking, erasing, and rescripting what your idea was to match the perfection that was created in their perspective of your growth.

Let's stop it right here. You are at the *RED* light in traffic because you had a conference meeting with someone who was not invited to the level-up experience. Therefore, you could consider what was shared but remember your limits are boundless when you truly trust and believe. As well as activating with clarity. Look at both scripts and come up with one. If it is helpful to you, take a moment to look at the voices and contributions that you have received and then compare them to your original list. Choose and consolidate both what you will proceed with caution and activate in your steps. You can proceed when you trust. The collaboration is helpful but can be fuel for a distraction to keep us with the lizard brain going back and forth. This makes our goals seem further and further away and become unrealistic because we have entered the playground of second-guessing ourselves and the anxiety playground that has taken over.

Effective leaders are disruptors. When they find the nugget that has them at the red light of being innovative and rewarded, they activate what is necessary to level up. The behavior and action to pause is a learned behavior that continues to surface because you have not fully released what you have survived and given yourself access to growing. You are no longer that person from the "survival narrative"—you have broken away.

In activation, it will not always be a perfect response but it will be a forward movement toward the overarching goals and your personal development success. Have you ever met PERFECT? If yes, at what cost to your emotional wellness, wealth, and esteem?

Anxiety beyond the diagnosis is a behavior. Behavior has a function and/or purpose to avoid or to get which one is driving you in your daily decisions in relationships, career, and leadership. Which one would you like to activate?

Motivated by DISAPPOINTMENT and ANGER

Are you serving your *LOWER* self and **lowered motivation**? Your lower self has been violated, overlooked, passed over, non-committed, and inconsistent. When you are captured by a history of who you were versus who you are becoming, you remain stuck and confused. Telling yourself you are not deserving—don't have time. No one will want what you offer and have chest pain, fatigue, and a foggy brain. You would need to unlearn all of these downloads and clear your emotional cookies (like the computer cookies) from your career bandwidth.

Starting the challenging conversation. Have you done an inventory of your true and confirmed contributions to the team and conversation? What is your authentic awareness meter in knowing your value with the unlearning process while you build your confidence, and esteem and strut your stuff? You have been certified and credentialed. Beyond the social expectations to qualify you, are you aware of the internal struggle or gifted design that you bring to every experience? Do you believe it? If you have doubt, please confront yourself and tell yourself why.

People are betting on you remaining silent and betting on your silence to go along to get along. People, and more importantly **YOU, WIN** when you are no longer silent and ignoring the hidden treasures within. It is not to suggest that you need to confront it by going through the weeds of therapy to level up. However, let's name the conflict (internal/external) so that you can engage in your mourning and grief and be able to access the tools within that will shift your manifestation of resentment, anger, and loss to the power and influence you have with the WINS gained in each iteration of your growth.

The challenge before you now is that you have become more clear in learning that some of the experiences that you have tucked away have prepared you for this very moment of leveling up your career. Your experiences are your experiences. Some carry an emotional and physical weight that keeps you waiting at the **RED LIGHT** for permission to move forward. The longer that it can keep you feeling "played and ignored" the longer it has captured your attention from what you have gained. As long as you choose to sit in the manifestation and not allow yourself to release the negative feelings and thoughts that can be found in the weeds—you will feel limited in your ability to be the effective and qualified CEO in your life.

SILENCE season is over! Let's confront what we need to confront and empower our voices so that we can level up across all of the intersections that life yields. When we open ourselves to the opportunities of what these situations can bring we are **SURVIVING**—gifting us with strength, resilience, and insight—then we are positioned for our GREATNESS and able to recognize that we hold the keys to what limits us. And that is not a glass ceiling that keeps us from being SNATCHED.

LET'S GET SNATCHED...

You have experienced this chapter and hopefully had some revelations. In your role as a leader, are you collaborative or in competition with old values? Have you been able to see some of the limiting beliefs that guide you to the blind spots and roadblocks that exist? Are you ready to activate the daily divorce of self that will identify what you would benefit from unlearning and shifting your leadership practices? That is truly the authentic activation in practice with the appropriate strategy.

Getting SNATCHED is the activation of working within the perspective of change with the **S**trategic **N**etworking and **A**lliances yield **T**ransformative **C**ollaborations that **H**elp **E**nergize **D**evelopment. Transformation guides us to constantly invest in how we grow through one experience to the next while building bridges in our leadership.

The best value and investment in self is to activate the change and divorce the habits that have you repeating the patterns and not valuing your skill set.

When you remember and confidently believe you are who you say you are the competition is over, and you don't have to prove it to others.

How do you learn to LIVE in your TRUTH?

Walking in your purpose, claiming victory and promotion?

Be strategic and gain clarity in your focus to get the GEMS of life and SHIFT from Survivor to LEVEL UP with EXCELLENCE.

In my work with many professionals who are striving to level up, the conversation of survival seems to always rise to the top. It is the experience that most individuals are unaware of what they are carrying in their energy while communicating. This impact causes you to have various false starts where you are working on promotion, pay increase, and simply leveling up to CEO with holes in your plan. In the course of the 15+ years of doing the work, it has become clear that a new BLUEPRINT or GPS route is needed. It takes a perspective of work that rolling up the sleeves becomes the game changer that silence was keeping you away from. As well as a true investment in a mindset shift that develops value of you knowing that, to create the wellness balance of work-life harmony, something external is needed to address the internal dialogue.

If you are truly ready to expedite the activation in practice, it is a seamless decision to reflect on how you can grow, develop, and secure the desired position that you have been seeking all of this time.

When you consider what the framework and formula of the GPS opens up it reveals

- **Not only** the ability to identify **GOALS**
- **Not only** the ability to identify the **PLAN**
- **Not only** the ability to identify the **STRATEGY**

But it also identifies the *BLIND SPOTS* and *BARRIERS* that are keeping you from what it is that you want and provides you the side-by-side support of what is needed to work through them because you are going to need some guided accountability.

When you are truly positioning yourself for leveling up to **CEO** status and beyond, this **BLUEPRINT** becomes the effective side-by-side strategy that will guide you there. You will no longer feel and/or experience being passed over when the promotion has been well deserved and earned by you.

Get started and secure your discovery breakthrough today!

Choose to level up your leadership and create the life that you want to lead and live on your own terms.

Questions for Reflection

1. What is important to you when setting your professional/personal goals?
2. How do you view your pathway in leadership from the start of your career to where you would identify reaching your optimal success?
3. Have you been guided to explore to learn more about themes that have elevated or stunted your progress in Leadership/Business?
4. How do you view the importance of your development as a professional in leadership beyond a workshop or brief retreat?
5. What transactional plan of action would you need to confront the conflict/collaboration of your leadership's current strategy?

8 So... It's a Sex Podcast?

Dr. Sara Vogel

"So... it's a sex podcast," my husband said definitively.

"No, it's more than that. It's about women finding their personal power and agency. We just happen to talk about sex... well... a lot," I clarified.

"Sex pod," he joked.

~~~~~~

Okay, okay, so I started a sex podcast. But it needed to be done. And I would argue that if you are working in sexual education and consulting, you should start one, too. I'll explain this shortly, but before I do, let me explain how I got here.

From Higher Education to an LLC

For over 15 years, I have worked as a higher education administrator building inclusive communities where all students feel valued and accepted for who they are. For the last six years, I have worked specifically as a Title IX Coordinator addressing allegations of sexual harassment, sexual assault, dating and domestic violence, and stalking. Through my work, I have supported hundreds of survivors of sexual assault, relationship violence, and stalking. I have become incredibly comfortable working in uncomfortable spaces, especially as it relates to navigating the complex scenarios including sexual coercion, sexual harassment, and sexual assault. As a Title IX Coordinator, I conduct preventative education on consent, sexual communication, and how to establish sexual boundaries. Although my favorite part of the job is educating our communities about how to engage in healthy sexual relationships, the majority of my time is spent on administrative investigations after allegations of gender-based violence are reported. This work is heartbreaking and often ends with a resolution that does not feel fair for any of the parties involved.

Witnessing and listening to the trauma, rage, and pain inflicted on parties, I began to question—what are we doing as a society to prevent these situations from occurring? Were school systems helping young people understand the dynamics of healthy intimate relationships? Were colleges and universities

DOI: 10.4324/9781003314660-8

giving their students the tools to communicate their sexual values and boundaries and honor their sexual agency? The answer was a resounding no.

The non-existent sexual education pipeline of the United States has left people in intimate situations they are unprepared to handle physically, emotionally, and spiritually. With the students I worked with, they often reported feeling immense pressure to perform sexually, yet lacked basic knowledge of how their sexual bodies and minds worked. They could not understand their desires, and more importantly, how to give and ask for affirmative and enthusiastic consent before and during sexual encounters. Most of the time, students I helped were reconciling the immense shame they felt around their bodies and sexualities, and had no clue how to have nuanced conversations with their partners about their sexual needs, desires, and boundaries. Although this was not the sole reason for sexual and intimate partner violence, it became a large part of my conversations with students. Students craved education on sex and intimacy agency, yet our school systems and educators were unable to provide this education.

It has been an honor to support sexual assault survivors, but the question of preventative education continued to nag at me. I could not shake my desire to be doing more to increase preventative education, in the hopes that I may be able to normalize conversations on sex, increase sexual confidence in others, and give them the tools to navigate sexual situations. I wanted to host authentic, and often difficult, conversations about sex, sexual identities, sexual communication, as a different avenue to curb sexual assault and intimate partner violence. These ponderings became the foundation from which I would build my Ladybits and Leadership, LLC. It took around three-and-a-half years of dreaming about this work, researching the market for comprehensive sexual education programs, ideating what my ideal business would look like, and making some key connections with business mentors, to feel comfortable enough to register Ladybits and Leadership, LLC in January 2022.

Exploring the Sexual Education and Empowerment Pipeline

Any good business fills a void missing in the community, or approaches an existing problem with a new solution. When I looked at the void of sexual empowerment education and the comprehensive sexual education pipeline in the United States of America, the outlook was bleak—it was essentially non-existent. According to the Guttmacher Institute (2023), only 38 states and the District of Columbia mandate sex education; only 11 states require consent to be part of this conversation. Where schools require this education, families still have the option to opt out and shield their children from these important lessons (Guttmacher Institute, 2023). There is not only a lack of formal education on sex and sexuality, the United States is also witnessing a fervent effort from certain states to ban books that include topics on gender identity and queer theory, narratives, and education. The American Library Association reported that in 2022, efforts to ban books from school libraries doubled from the previous years, and amounted to the highest number of complaints the Association received in the 20 years they have been tracking this data (Alter & Harris, 2023). Due to the lack of public education on this topic, it has been left to private, independent businesses to fill the sexual education void as a means to create an informed and empowered citizenry.

When I reflect on my own personal journey of learning about my sexuality, I too, experienced a lack of education both in the home and school. The week of sexual education I received in public school during my seventh-grade wellness class, was approached through a fear-based model of teaching that focused on anatomy, STIs, and pregnancy. We looked at 2-D models of vulvas, vaginas, penises, and scrotums. There was no discussion of the variety of sizes, colors, and shapes of these body parts to normalize that we all look a little different. There were no nuanced discussions about how we felt about our genitals or our sexual identities. Birth control methods only included the pill and condoms, and abortions were not discussed. We did not discuss consent or how strong sexual communication can help individuals draw boundaries with a partner or partners. The week of education ended with pictures of sexually transmitted infections in advanced stages, and a video of a vaginal birth. Sex was posited as something to figure out at a later time, ideally when we were adults and married in a heterosexual relationship.

Never in the conversation did we talk about pleasure or consent being critical for healthy sexual relationships. Nor was the teacher able or prepared to discuss the intersections of a person's moral and ethical values, trauma, and the confusing societal norms regarding sex in this discussion. The teacher taught the bare minimum required by law, and moved on to the easier conversations of wellness including career planning and selecting which co-curricular activities we would participate in during high-school. Although, this chapter is not about the failures of our society to teach people about sexual health and wellness, I thought it important to share some personal experiences and data as a way to demonstrate how society fails young people (or any people for that matter) by not providing them the knowledge and tools on building sexual confidence, advocating for their pleasure, understanding the diversity of sexual experiences, and how to communicate those sexual needs and wants with a partner.

When society provides policies and education that support inclusive, medically-accurate, sex-positive education on sexual identity and consent, violence rates decrease (UNESCO, 2018). Given the lack of sex education in the United States, and political and sociological division on the topic, I realized that if I wanted to be a part of the shift toward providing this much-needed education, I needed to be part of the change I wished to see in my lifetime. So, I began Ladybits and Leadership, LLC to fill this void of sexual education and build a groundswell movement in my community. Although I knew that education alone would not stop sexual violence from occurring, it would still help people unlearn the toxic messages they received about their bodies and sexual lives, and find tools and the confidence to take action toward living a more sexually empowered life. Together, little by little, my company's work could move us toward a more just and more empowered society.

Deciding to Take Bold Action to Start My Business

Armed with data and a personal passion for the topic, I asked myself, *"What kind of sexual education company should I build?"* As I was grappling with this question, one of my favorite podcasters, Cathy Heller, offered the opportunity for her listeners to learn how to create and monetize a podcast through her online course, *Your Turn to Podcast.* As a natural storyteller, and someone who has listened to hundreds of survivor stories, I knew this was the right direction for my business. It felt like a podcast would be the most fun and aligned way to begin a business.

As a doctorate student, I learned that some people believe the "best" and "most valid way" to "create knowledge" and "gain credibility" was through publishing original research in academic journals and presenting at well-known conferences. However, I also learned there is incredible value in narrative research, autoethnographies, and storytelling. As a Native Hawaiian woman, I understood the value of storytelling, as our cultural knowledge has been passed on through storytelling for hundreds of years. Neuroscience also shows that stories elicit greater comprehension and are more likely to change people's behavior (Renkin, 2020). Another reason I chose to share this sexual education through a global podcast was due to issues of equity and access. Not all people have the ability to access or read academic journals, research articles, or professional conferences. However, podcasts can be accessed for free via the Internet. In my opinion, hosting an educational podcast was the best way to disseminate powerful educational material to the greatest number of people possible.

As I thought about joining the podcasting program, the first issue was the cost of the program. The course cost $2,500 and I did not know how to tell my husband that I would be taking $2,500 from our savings account to pay for this course. I knew we had the money and that we could afford it. What held me back from telling him about this expenditure, was the thought of confessing to my husband that I wanted to eventually quit my secure job in student affairs, and become a business owner who runs educational initiatives around sex education and empowerment. My dream of being a business owner would eventually have huge ramifications for our financial well-being and overall stability. We had been together for over a decade and throughout our marriage, he supported me emotionally and financially through my Masters and Doctorate, moving all over the country, to support my dream to one day become a Vice-Chancellor of Student Affairs at a major university. Telling him I was "throwing away" this dream I worked toward my entire adult life, to "chase a new dream" felt like a betrayal to the sacrifices he and I made over the last decade together.

I struggled to find the courage and the words to describe my dreams for something bigger than a career in student affairs. So, I took the money from my personal account and did not tell him I was signing up for the class. I knew at some point I would have the courage to let him know I was taking the class and starting a podcast. It took a couple of months after the class began to have the idea solidified and the words needed to explain to him why I wanted to start my own business and the value of a podcast. More on this decision can be found later in this chapter.

Building a Business Mindset by Battling Imposter Syndrome

As I began the *Your Turn to Podcast* course, I quickly ran into imposter syndrome. Many women in particular struggle with the concept of imposter syndrome, and I was no exception to this. Imposter syndrome (originally "imposter phenomenon") was developed by psychologists Pauline Rose Clance and Suzanne Imes in 1978, after they explored the minds and actions of high-achieving women. Since then, there has been much research about the complexities of imposter syndrome and the connection between racism, classism, and other forms of systemic bias and discrimination (Tulshyan & Burey, 2021). During the podcasting course, I doubted my abilities, and messages of imposter syndrome ran through my head constantly. They sounded like:

- This is a ridiculous idea.
- People have tried to open a business like this and failed. You will be no different.
- This is a waste of time.
- You would be better-served staying in your lane in higher education.
- You are giving up a whole career for a dream that will go nowhere. How irresponsible.
- You are not qualified enough to start a business.
- You don't have the money or the time to begin a business.
- This is going to fail. You are going to fail. You are going to be a failure.

In order to combat these negative messages, it was incredibly helpful to participate in groups that focused on supporting new women business owners. There was a support group built into each podcasting class. Every week, Cathy hosted a class that focused both on building a business mindset which addressed imposter syndrome as well as other emotional and mental blocks, as well as some technical aspects of building a podcast, a brand, and a business. Together, in community, I, along with the other podcasting students, were able to hear positive and encouraging messages that gave us the confidence and drive needed to begin a podcast and business.

Start by Making it Messy

Cathy, our podcasting instructor, emphasized that the best way to combat imposter syndrome was to take small empowered actions every day. She called it "making it messy." What that meant was the best way to prove to yourself you could do something, and fight back against imposter syndrome, was to take small, messy, imperfect actions. For example, at the beginning of the podcasting course, she had students record the introduction to their podcast and post it on podcasting channels as well as on their social media or email lists. She gave us the guidance that an intro was to be between 1 and 2 minutes, introduce the themes of the podcast, and what people could expect when they listened to the podcast. When that assignment came out, my imposter syndrome said, "Your topic is too messy. You sound nasally when you record. You are not qualified to make a podcast about these topics." When I had these thoughts, I acknowledged them by telling myself, "I hear you, I acknowledge you, but I am just going to make it messy, anyway."

I spent hours writing the one-minute script, recorded it four times, edited the best version, told myself this is perfect for now, and then took brave action and published it online. In taking imperfect action, I not only chipped away at my imposter syndrome, I also solidified my podcasting and business idea. Additionally, I asserted to the world that I was a woman who was bold enough to create, edit, and publish a public, global podcast about sex, gender, and power.

Your Turn to Podcast offered weekly support groups that focused on the technical aspects of recording and publishing podcasts including microphone use, editing software, troubleshooting audio issues, and utilizing online podcasting platforms. During those meetings, we were able to take empowered, messy action, make mistakes, fix them, and grow together. This support-rich environment provided new business owners and podcasters like myself the assurance needed to take calculated risks, acknowledge that failures are a part of the process, and realize that should you have a question, there was always someone in the group who had an answer. I credit the supportive environment that Cathy and her team provided for setting us up for success. As we moved through the course, my messy action continued, and as a result, my confidence grew. I found myself becoming bolder and more confident in my actions, and able to take on new challenges. My internal voice began to shift, and I changed my language from "I am trying to be a business owner," to, "I am a business owner," and from, "I am trying to start a podcast," to "I host a podcast." After starting my podcasting class in October 2021, by January 2022, I had registered my business, Ladybits and Leadership, LLC and in February 2022, I posted my first episode which was distributed world-wide through Apple Podcasts, Spotify, and Google Podcasts. Ladybits and Leadership: The Podcast had gone global.

The Value of a Podcast in Building Connection and Empathy

Ladybits and Leadership, is both the name of my business and podcast, and speaks to the connection between a woman's/female-identified individual's most intimate parts (physical, mental, and emotional) and her ability to lead or hold power. Due to decades of racism, misogyny, and patriarchy, women are socialized to experience and hold shame around their bodies, sexuality, and motherhood. It is my belief that until women can unlearn the shame around their ladybits (whatever that looks like for them) they cannot fully step into their power. But where do women go to talk about these deeply held beliefs of shame and disempowerment? What spaces exist for them to hear from one another about healing from sexual violence, process common issues of sexual harassment, commiserate on the difficulties of being a new mom, or learn how to love their bodies? The answer, according to Dr. Brene Brown, author of *Women and Shame: Reaching Out, Speaking Truths and Building Connection* (2004), says very few of these spaces exist in the world today, and in order for women to move out of shame, they must build empathy. My goal with Ladybits and Leadership: The Podcast, was to use humor, authentic dialogue, and candor to talk about the difficult topics of womanhood, so that participants could learn about socialized shame, build empathy, find connection, and restructure how they view their bodies, sexuality, and motherhood.

On the podcast, I have covered topics including: surviving sexual harassment and assault, getting an abortion, vaginal health, childfree/childless lives, sexual attraction, menstrual cycles, single motherhood, pregnancy loss, body image, fatness, queerness, and experiences with pedophilia, postpartum depression, menopause, and addressing mental and physical wellness after trauma. The education I provide through Ladybits and Leadership, centers around sex, power, relationships, trauma, harm, and healing. These are all incredibly complex and difficult topics that require time and space to unpack, therefore, the long-form podcast is a wonderful venue to build an intimate space for guests to share their personal stories, and for the listeners to participate in this learning in a space where they felt most comfortable. A podcast allows a person to explore their learning, and resulting thoughts or feelings in a private way where there is no threat of safety, nor potential to be shamed publicly.

The Power of Podcasts as a Business Tool

Podcasts are quickly becoming a new way for people to connect with others, and can serve as an incredibly powerful learning and business building tool. According to groups like Edison Research (2022), who run media surveys regarding the state of podcasting both in the USA and globally, there are many indicators that podcasting is continuing to grow as a powerful information sharing and business development and advertising platform. Eighty-eight percent of Americans own a smartphone, and therefore have access to free podcast platforms such as Apple Podcasts, Spotify, and Google Podcasts. Currently, over one-third of Americans (approximately 104 million people) listen to podcasts regularly, and during the COVID-19 pandemic, podcasting listenership grew. Sixty-two percent of the US population aged 12 and over have listened to a podcast and over 75% of US citizens are familiar with what a podcast is (Buzzsprout, 2023).

Podcasts are a great way for businesses to connect with their current and potential customers, as well as help customers understand their business from a deeper, emotional level. Data shows that when customers make a purchase, they rely on the know-like-trust funnel, which means customers are more likely to do business with companies that provide quality content and provide a solution (Stanly, 2022). Audio platforms provide a new venue for business owners, particularly sex educators, to build a know-like-trust purchase funnel with customers, as it allows them the opportunities to provide important education and tools.

Sexual health education is currently a popular topic of interest on many podcasts, and some sex educators have made this the entire focus of their podcasts. Here are examples of the sex education podcasts that are often listed in the top of the charts:

- Sex with Emily, with Sex Therapist, Dr. Emily Morse.
- Sexology, with Dr. Nazanin Moali.
- Sex and Psychology, with Dr. Justin Lehmiller.
- The Sensual Self Podcast, with sexuality doula, Ev'Yan Whitney.
- The Authentic Sex Podcast, with tantric practitioner and sexologist Juliet Allen.
- Sex with Dr. Jess, with Dr. Jessica O'Reilly.
- Where Should We Begin, with Esther Perel.

Podcasts are not only great ways to build a customer base for one's sexual education business, but they also help democratize sexual education. In a world that continues to see high rates of sexual and relationship violence, sexual shame, and trauma, one could make an ethical argument that we need as many sex educators as possible creating podcasts to help educate and empower the population about sexual agency, power dynamics, and how to address situations and systems of violence.

Podcasts do not require the listener to have reading skills in order to learn the information being provided, therefore, this opens up the information to larger groups of diverse listeners. Additionally, this information can be consumed anywhere, as listeners can consume the information in a car on their commutes, while working out at the gym, or cooking dinner. This ability to multitask while learning via podcast differentiates podcasts from books or online articles. Podcasts also take less time and energy to produce than academic or research articles, yet can still be researched-based and provide empirical knowledge. Further, listeners do not need to have access to academic databases in order to access this research. One can download a podcast for free, therefore, podcasts are not cost-prohibitive. Last, the digital nature of podcasts allows listeners to easily share the link to the podcasts via text, social media, or email—increasing the likelihood that more people will get access to this important information. One of my goals with Ladybits and Leadership was to help educate as many people as possible about their power and agency in their intimate lives, therefore a podcast was a perfect place to begin as it allowed me to disseminate my message and information to a global audience of potentially eight billion listeners.

Preparing to Host a Sex Podcast

Due to the amount of trauma often associated with topics of sexuality, bodily autonomy, power, and agency, I had to ensure I was as informed and safe as possible when addressing these topics with the podcast guests, as well as with my own experiences. When I took stock of what preparation I completed in my professional work as a Title IX Coordinator, and in my academic doctoral research on power and gender, I found enough evidence to demonstrate I was equipped to host this podcast. What I did not expect was the emotional journey I would experience by confronting my own unresolved trauma regarding my body and my experiences with sexual harassment. Hosting this podcast became the impetus to continue my healing and liberation journey, as well as helping others do the same.

Dealing with My Own Trauma

Research demonstrates that 81% of women experience some form of sexual harassment (Chattergee, 2018) during their lifetime. Situations include sexual comments, unwanted sexual touching, and sexual assault in various spaces including public spaces, online, and/or at work. To prepare for this podcast, I reflected on all the ways I experienced the spectrum of violence as a woman. I completed these reflective exercises through therapy, speaking with my partner, and doing countless hours of personal development such as journaling and researching. Being immersed in this work, I found that the pain from my experiences with sexual violence and trauma were more profound and present than I realized. As I began to design topics for future podcast conversations, I found I still needed to grieve and process my sexual- and body-related trauma. Only by doing this necessary pre-work, was I able to freely share my truth, take risks, and be vulnerable.

As I reflected on the sexual situations I have experienced, I began to find evidence of sexual harassment across my lifespan. Those who work in sexual education and sexual violence prevention work will inevitably begin to reflect on their lives and, at times, will uncover examples of experienced trauma, that would be beneficial to confront in order to best serve clients. For me, it was important to process my experiences, so I could tell those stories on coercion and consent with courage. Navigating what topics to disclose of one's personal experience to a public audience is an art, and I needed to make sure I had done the work to understand why I was sharing this trauma with them, what purpose would it serve, and to understand if I was okay with the emotional cost it would take on my mental health and wellness.

Navigating Shared Trauma and Personal Boundaries

In addition to sharing personal trauma I experienced, there were other stories of body trauma I wanted to share, but they included other people. This added a new element to my preparation and pre-work, as I needed to connect with those who shared in this trauma. One clear example of this was my abortion story. Although this unintended pregnancy was *my* experience, it was also an experience I shared with my husband. In order to ethically share our experience publicly, I felt it right to discuss with him why I wished to share the story, what good it could bring to the audience, and discuss the potential consequences that he and I may face due to the disclosure. Together we had to navigate difficult conversations about our individual feelings and emotions about this experience—something that at the time of the abortion, was not done due to an immense amount of shame I felt when this occurred. Working through this shared trauma proved to be more difficult than I originally believed it would be, as it brought up our differing fundamental beliefs on how public one should be with their sex lives and trauma.

My husband is an incredibly private person which is the polar opposite to my natural inclination to be open and public about my life and opinions. Therefore, when I decided I would be going to take my advocacy for sexual empowerment to the next level by hosting a global podcast focused on storytelling where I often refer to my individual and partnered sexual experiences, we disagreed fundamentally on the extent of what needed to be shared. It was not an easy time in our relationship, but with open communication about intent, goals, and boundaries, he and I managed to find a place where we understood where the privacy boundaries were as it related to our marriage and raising a son. Although this podcast and business were my own, it was critical to have these conversations during the planning and early implementation phase of the podcast to ensure that I knew how to remain respectful of my family's boundaries as I moved forward.

Some of the questions we needed to navigate as a couple included:

- What topics was he comfortable with me speaking about?
- What conversations was he less comfortable with me speaking about?
- What topics were absolutely off limits?
- How would we handle privacy issues if this podcast were to gain momentum and have thousands (or millions) of downloads?

- How would we handle speaking with our parents and friends about the podcast?
- Would you want to listen to the podcast before it aired?
- Would he want to be on the podcast?

In May 2022, when the world learned that the Supreme Court of the United States intended to overturn *Roe v. Wade*, eliminating a national protection for abortion rights, I made the decision that I needed to use my voice and platform to share my abortion experience. When I experienced an abortion a decade earlier, I felt an incredible amount of loneliness and shame. I lived with that shame for over a decade, and swore my husband to secrecy due to my shame. This shame affected my life for years. In this time of political and social unrest, I wanted to humanize the issue of abortion, and assure those going through an abortion, or had experienced an abortion, that their reason to terminate a pregnancy was valid and that they were not alone. If Ladybits and Leadership was to promote liberation from shame and encourage people to find their voice, power, and agency, then I needed to model the way. By the time I recorded my abortion episode, I had had many conversations with both my husband and my therapist. I was ready. We as a couple were ready.

Business owners who share their authentic lives through global podcasts will find that it is incredibly important to be on the same page with one's intimate partner and other close family members because, inevitably, their lives, experiences, and feelings will be entangled in the stories told. In addition to speaking about this topic with my husband, I also shared my decision to talk about my abortion with my parents and in-laws before posting the episode. Never before had I shared this information with them, and the disclosure was incredibly difficult emotionally. By coming to them privately, and answering any questions they had about the procedure or about my reason for talking about it on the podcast, I was able to help them understand why I chose to share this story. It was critical for my family to understand that I was not sharing my trauma for sharing sake—it was a way for me to use my lived experience to validate for another listener that they are not alone.

By sharing my conflicting emotions about my abortion, how I reconciled my trauma, what resources I turned to, and how I worked through trauma in a healthy way, gave listeners who may be silently suffering, and feeling alone, the tools needed to do the healing on their own. I held my breath as I pressed post on my abortion story. After living for years in silent shame, struggling alone to make meaning of the experience, my truth was now free in a global way. The influx of messages of support, love, and "me too" messages were astounding. So many of my friends (some of them in their 40s and 50s) shared that they too had experienced an abortion and lived with their shame and secrecy for years. For some of them, I was the first person they shared this with. Liberating my story, helped others liberate themselves.

Weeks after I posted the abortion story, I received a message from an unknown person in South Africa who said she listened to my abortion podcast after searching for episodes on abortion. She shared she had just had a surgical abortion and was struggling to make meaning of it. This woman knew she was not ready to have a child, and her boyfriend was giving her grief for choosing an abortion. After listening to my abortion episode, she felt compelled to reach out to me personally to gain more insight as to how I made that decision and how long it took me to emotionally heal from it. When she asked me via Instagram message how long it would take until she "healed" emotionally from the experience, I was honest with her and told her I was still healing. I emphasized that I never wanted to be placed in a position of needing an abortion, but it happened and I made the best decision for me at the time, and assured her that at the time, she made the best decision for her and her life, as well. We were able to converse through instant messenger and I was able to offer support, resources, encouragement, and love. This is the power of podcasting. One never knows who is listening or from where. Sometimes by sharing a personal truth, one may just be saving another's life halfway across the world.

As Ladybits and Leadership—the podcast and business continues to grow, I will continue to navigate difficult conversations with people I know and love, supporters and detractors alike. When my toddler son comes of age, should he want to listen to my podcast, I will have to be prepared to answer the questions he may have. Speaking about sex and our bodily autonomy should not be controversial, and yet, that is the reality of the world today. The only way to continue to move the needle forward in gender equity, sexual education, and reproductive justice, is to create the spaces to share stories and discuss the complexities of these difficult subjects.

Coming out to my Workplace

The other entity I needed to share my new business and podcast with was my place of employment. At the time that I began my business, I worked as a Title IX Coordinator at a public college. In my role, I am expected to conduct fair, timely, impartial investigations. When I registered my business, I reached out to my place of employment to submit the paperwork needed to disclose my business and understand the rules and regulations about any potential conflicts of interest in the future. There were many people that worked for the public university and had businesses on the side. I did not believe there would be any issues, as I had a strong understanding of these matters. However, shortly after my first episode was published, I was told by a colleague that a male colleague had listened to my podcast and was concerned that I would not be able to conduct my role as a Title IX Coordinator in a fair and impartial way, due to me hosting conversations on self-pleasure and masturbation. Stunned that this instructor did not see the connection between sexual education and sexual violence, I addressed this concern directly on my podcast. I waited for a formal complaint to arrive from this colleague, but none came. It is important that those who work full-time, in addition to beginning their sexual education business, understand the rules and policies around secondary employment. It would be advantageous to inform one's direct supervisor about this additional employment to ensure that rules are being followed. Additionally, a supervisor may be able to help navigate the politics of a work environment, should rumors or complaints in the workplace begin.

Unexpected Beautiful Things

Since launching the podcast in February 2022, I have posted 35 episodes online and have accumulated over 5,000 downloads. The podcast has not only helped me launch my business and assert myself as an expert in the field of sexual education, it has also created a strong know-like-trust funnel where potential clients who listen to the podcast reach out to me to inquire about my services. Due to my experience as a podcaster and sex educator, I have been hired by colleges and universities to present on topics covered in the podcast including: women in business, the importance of diverse voices in media, and sexual pleasure and consent. The podcast has given me stronger reasons to connect with other sex educators in the field, interview them, and build a network of support and resources. The field of sex education is small, and the networking opportunities from podcasting is immense and will move your forward in your understanding of the field and the various approaches to this work,

Although the business momentum is promising, the real celebration is in the way these episodes have impacted the guests and listeners. It has opened space for individuals to begin the healing processes around the shame and trauma of their bodies. Nothing delights me more than listeners sending me pictures of their first vibrators, sharing their successes as they become more confident in their sex lives and bodies, signing up for individual and couples' therapy, and having open conversations with their doctors to ask about menstrual cycles and birth control options. People have begun to question toxic thought patterns, societal standards and norms, and evaluate the way they show up in relationships. This critical thinking has led them to take action to care for themselves and others. This was the vision for Ladybits and Leadership—to bring healing and empowerment around bodies, sexual identities, and sexual lives, and the podcast and business are accomplishing this. Additionally, as the podcast grows in listenership, opportunities for business contracts to educate outside the podcast are increasing monthly. What began as a dream, has not only turned into a reality, but a profitable one at that.

Belief in your Ability to Learn

As a relatively new business owner, I have had many, many experiences to learn from as I began my podcast and business. Above are examples of lessons learned about the podcasting process. Below I share my greatest business takeaways in the hope that readers may find the courage and scrappiness to begin where they are. More diverse voices are needed desperately in the podcasting space, and by making the work lucrative, will ensure that diverse voices will continue to add toward the collective knowledge within sexual education.

Courage as a Business Mindset

At the start, I knew nothing about beginning a business. I did not come from a family of entrepreneurs. I did not know any entrepreneurs in my immediate circles of friends. My first exposure to beginning my own business was through my podcasting course. Our podcasting instructor, Cathy Heller, reminded us over and over again, that there was no right path and right way to begin a business. She offered to us the belief that once we get courageous and take messy action, that the business confidence would follow. And that is exactly what happened—I took messy action, and little by little, success by success, I began to embody a business owner. "I am thinking about hosting a podcast," evolved into "I am trying to start a podcast," which changed into, "I have a podcast published online," which then became, "I am a podcaster." Business owners must develop a courageous mindset to begin taking the little actions that will lead to a strong business mindset. Once that confidence in self is developed, bigger risks and bigger rewards can be gleaned—but it all begins with small courageous steps.

Scrappiness and Resourcefulness Reign Supreme

The next lesson I learned from beginning my sexual education business and podcast, was that a business owner's ability to get scrappy and resourceful, is one of the greatest emotional assets. When a business owner is scrappy, they are not worried about perfectionism, which is often the enemy of progress, they are just worried about getting the job done. As one endeavors on a new journey such as entrepreneurship, the goal is to keep progressing toward the dream, using the resources they have at their disposal. As a new entrepreneur, Googling, "How to…" was an everyday experience. I still turn to Google as my biggest business instructor—how to record a podcast, how to post a podcast online, how to transcribe a podcast, how to design a business card, how to create a business contract or invoice, how to file business taxes.

Podcasts hosted by female entrepreneurs became a massive part of my learning as a first-time business owner. My goal was to listen to as many diverse voices as possible, to gain insight into building a business mindset, marketing and social media strategies, developing online educational courses, and branding and growth. My favorites included: The Cathy Heller Show with Cathy Heller, I am Your Korean Mom with Simone Grace Seol, Online Marketing Made Easy with Amy Porterfield, Hello Seven Podcast with Rachel Rodgers, Make Money as a Life Coach with Stacey Boehman, and The Jasmine Star Show with Jasmine Star. I joked with people that through my podcasts, I was getting a free MBA, but in reality, they were opening my eyes to the various systems at play when one is beginning a business.

Last, I joined a virtual network of women entrepreneurs called Launch Your Fempire, by Aesha Shapiro, a business incubator which focused on helping women develop and launch their businesses. Although this resource was not free, it was a solid business investment as every week we learned from other women entrepreneurs about building a business model, pricing our services, collaborating with brands, developing brand collateral, managing finances, and more. At the end of the year, we were required to launch a product or project. It was the impetus I needed to make big business moves and put my offers out there. Meeting once a week virtually with other women who were also in the beginning stages of their business development, gave me the opportunity to discuss business issues and get real-time coaching from my peers and the mentors of the program. I was able to network and find support and resources and vendors they vetted and trusted, and, more importantly, helped me feel less alone in this entrepreneurship journey. Through the business network, I shared my successes, no matter how big or small, and immediately received the positive support needed to persist in entrepreneurship, especially when mistakes occurred, or my belief in myself waned. We spoke about the complexities of being women in the business world, and for many of us, the complexities of managing motherhood and business. Entrepreneurship can be a lonely space. When one is a solo business owner, most of the thousands of business decisions made weekly rely on one's own intuition, education, and acumen. Even with a supportive partner or family, it can be a lonely, confusing space. Surrounding oneself with people in a similar situation, and mentors or coaches, will help an entrepreneur move farther, faster.

Deep Understanding of Trauma Cultivates Success and Longevity

When working in the field of sexual education, confronting trauma is inevitable. If one has not processed their own sexual trauma, it would be advantageous to do so to have the mental and emotional stamina to complete this work on a daily basis. If one has not taken coursework on trauma and its effect on the brain and body, it would be of benefit to do so. An unexpected benefit of this work, was diving into the research of sexual harassment, discrimination from a historical, gendered, sociological, religious, and cultural perspective. Having a stronger understanding of the factors that play a role in high rates of sexual violence, helped me understand and process my own experiences with these phenomena. The research I conducted, along with the somatic healing and therapeutic interventions, has not only made me feel more whole, and stronger, but also gave me the mental fortitude needed to address sexual trauma daily without experiencing vast amounts of vicarious trauma.

Make Business Joyful

Beginning a podcast and a business is incredibly hard work. As a new entrepreneur, one generally must be all the things for the business and podcast—the researcher, the administrative assistant, the editor, the marketing manager, the accountant, and the CEO. If joy is not present in the business building and maintenance it will be incredibly easy for a business owner to burn out. Therefore, my final piece of advice would be to keep joy at the forefront of business planning and development. What does this look like in practical terms? I start by asking myself, "Does this feel good? Does this business decision or direction feel good to me? Does it feel aligned with my skills, abilities, and ease? What does my body say about this decision? Do I need to be doing this all right now, or might it be better to do less, and move a little slower to bring ease and joy back into my life?" There have been several moments in building the business when I felt like my business decisions were out of alignment with intuition and my inner knowing, and this caused stress, worry, and dis-ease. When this occurred, I did not look forward to working on the business and the podcast, because the joy had been sucked out. When I lost sight of joy, I began to avoid my business and question if it was right for me to be an entrepreneur at all. When that occurred, I took stock of what was causing me trepidation or did not feel good, and asked myself, "What would a more joyful approach look like?" The moment to pause and reflect on what I really wanted for the business, and return to my gut instincts was what allowed me to move forward with joy and curiosity and excitement and avoid being caught in fear and unease and indecision and emotional pain. Joy allowed me to return back to the reason I wanted to begin the business in the first place—to help people cultivate delight and empowerment in their bodies and sexual lives.

Questions for Reflection

Podcasts take time, consistency, a vision, the ability to make it messy, and joy. They are a body of work that an entrepreneur can use to establish expertise in a field, and also be a space where a business owner can explore topics that delight and intrigue them. One who begins a sexual education podcast not only teaches others about the world of sexual empowerment, but also continues their own learning and reflection along the way. In this way, a podcast can serve both as a product to offer to customers, and also a tool for personal and professional development for the entrepreneur.

As this chapter concludes, I offer some questions for reflection for one to use to decide if beginning a podcast is the best move for their journey in entrepreneurship. I look forward to seeing your podcast and to you adding your voice to the symphony of sexual empowerment education.

Podcast Ideation

In order to stay committed to the joy of podcasting, it is important to explore what a dream podcast would look like.

Questions for Reflection:

- In what ways may you be able to translate your sexual education business into a podcast?
- Are there niche topics or perspectives as they relate to sexual education that you could speak about for hours?
- Would you prefer a solo podcast where it is just you teaching, speaking, bringing awareness to a topic? Or would it feel better to have guests? If you want to invite guests, who would be some guests that could speak on your topic?
- Do you prefer short or long podcasts? Would you want your podcast to be on-going or a limited series with different topics every season?
- Solo podcasts or would you want to have guests? Or a mix of the two?

Personal Disclosure

Podcasting is a very intimate form of sharing knowledge, and often involves sharing one's own experiences to build intimacy with the guest and the listeners.

Questions for Reflection:

- Have you decided which personal opinions and sexual experiences you are comfortable sharing with listeners?
- Are there others who may be impacted by you sharing these stories publicly that you may need to check in with before sharing these stories?
- How might you bring awareness to/ask permission of the folks who have shared stories with you?

Understanding of Sexual Trauma

When working in sexual education, it is common for one to feel triggered due to previous experiences with trauma.

Questions for Reflection

1. In what ways have you addressed your own experiences with sexual trauma?
2. Is there still more work that you could participate in to feel prepared to address others' sexual trauma when working in sexual education and podcasting?
3. Do you have a support network and/or support plan on how to address trauma when it arises during the podcasting process?

References

Alter, A., & Harris, E. A. (March 23, 2023). Attempts to Ban Books Doubled in 2022. *New York Times*. https://www.nytimes.com/2023/03/23/books/book-ban-2022.html?smid=url-share

Brown, B. (2004). *Women and Shame: Reaching Out, Speaking Truths, and Finding Connection*. 3C Press. ISBN 0975425234, 9780975425237

BuzzSprout. (March 7, 2023). Podcasts Statistics and Data. https://www.buzzsprout.com/blog/podcast-statistics##how-popular-are-podcasts

Chattergee, R. (February 21, 2018). A New Survey Finds 81 Percent Of Women Have Experienced Sexual Harassment. https://www.npr.org/sections/thetwo-way/2018/02/21/587671849/a-new-survey-finds-eighty-percent-of-women-have-experienced-sexual-harassment

Edison Research. (March 23, 2022). The Infinite Dial. https://www.edisonresearch.com/the-infinite-dial-2022/

Guttmacher Institute. (2023). Sex and HIV Education March 1, 2023. https://www.guttmacher.org/state-policy/explore/sex-and-hiv-education

Renkin, E. (April 11, 2020). How Stories Connect and Persuade Us: Unleashing The Brain Power Of Narrative. https://www.npr.org/sections/health-shots/2020/04/11/815573198/how-stories-connect-and-persuade-us-unleashing-the-brain-power-of-narrative

Stanly, J. (November 19, 2022). 3 Key Secrets To Building the Know, Like, And Trust Factor In Today's Digital Economy. https://www.entrepreneur.com/en-au/growth-strategies/3-key-secrets-to-building-the-know-like-and-trust-factor/439535

Tulshyan, R., & Burey, J. (February 11, 2021). Stop Telling Women They Have Imposter Syndrome. *Harvard Business Review.* https://hbr.org/2021/02/stop-telling-women-they-have-imposter-syndrome

UNESCO. (2018). International Technical Guide on Sexual Education: An Evidence-informed Approach. https://www.unaids.org/sites/default/files/media_asset/ITGSE_en.pdf

9 Developing Persona

Sex Therapist, Sex Professional, Sex Worker

Shanae Adams

Introduction

The business of sex is not a new phenomenon in the timeline of human history. Sex will always be a part of the human experience. Professionals in the business of sex are unique because they develop an intimate relationship with sexuality long before they get paid for it. My experience of living through sexuality with curiosity first makes me extremely angry at the systems that govern our society and disappointed in the access to comprehensive sexuality education. I am also sincere in pursuing the field and excited for what's next to come. My career development motto is "chase the dopamine." Neurodivergent in a neurotypical world dictated the need to understand my brain, motivations and give grace to functioning differently. Striking enough, I think my neurodivergence is a factor in my success as a student and an entrepreneur. "Findings indicate that for entrepreneurs with ADHD symptoms, entrepreneurial performance occurs when they simultaneously experience passion for founding and developing. This passion configuration is unique to successful ADHD-type entrepreneurs" (Hatak, 2021). I found the thing that gave me the warm tingles early in life and chased it into several dimensions of the business of sex. My ordeal is one of many journeys to success.

Sex Educator

Sexuality education came to me packaged in *Talk Sex* with Sue Johanson on late-night TV. Sue Johanson was a nurse turned sexuality educator. She pioneered the "Sunday Night Sex Show" on a rock radio station in 1984, and for 11 years, she had her own television show "Talk Sex" (Skuy, 1999). I stumbled upon something I did not know existed. Here was this old white woman talking about sex. She used figurines to show positions, had dildos all over her desk and people called in to talk to her. As I watched the show, I realized there was nothing Sue Johanson had that I didn't. All she did was deliver information to a camera that stimulated my curiosity. I decided I would have a show like that. I would be someone you could talk sex with.

DOI: 10.4324/9781003314660-9

I spread my newfound knowledge with my peers in school, and they were receptive to my information.

My gym teacher taught sex education at my school using the shock and awe technique with us. She showed pictures of sexually transmitted infections years into development and warned us that this would be our reality if we engaged in unprotected sex or in general. She also scared us into believing that masturbation was disgusting and perverted and that everyone would know if we engaged in such activities. We were shamed into not exploring our bodies and too overstimulated to ask questions. That didn't sit right with me. Sue never mentioned that STIs were the conclusion to expect when engaging in sex or that masturbation was harmful or shameful. Sue showed me what comprehensive sexuality education looked like and gave me a model to aspire to.

My mother was a sex-positive parent, although that is not the language she would use. She taught me how to read at a young age and surrounded me with sorites written by Black authors and books to provide information. One of my favorite books was *The Care and Keeping of You* by American Girls. This book was my first exposure to sex positivity. It was comprehensive, and its diagrams featured diverse body types, ethnicities, and body shapes. My mother was instrumental in helping me develop a healthy relationship with myself and affirming bodily autonomy. Through several books and teachings from my mother, I was able to grasp the notion of consent and that my body was mine and mine alone. I am grateful for my mother who helped me established sexual autonomy as a core of my identity and experience.

Between my private and public education, I used theatre to challenge my mind in novel ways. I loved that a good story transports the audience into unknown worlds. As an actor, I made those worlds come to life. Theatre brings community together on and off the stage. I witnessed the power of community in the braiding salon my mother owned. The beauty salon is sacred. The ritual of gender happens there. It was one of a few spots where I saw Black people lower their guards and be. Community felt warm and secure. I gravitated to spaces that made room for my whole self and experienced its healing and supporting nature. I learned how to encourage others through their accomplishments and failures. I held people through hard times and moments of joy. I taught and learned life skills that changed my points of view. Watching my community thrive moved me to aid in its growth.

Undergrad was the first time the profession of sexuality educator transitioned from fantasy to reality. The University of Missouri's Sexuality Health Advocate Peer Education (SHAPE) organization focused on developing and delivering sexuality education to campus students. This organization transfigured me. I received a trial by fire from my peers and began to build a vision of myself as a career sexuality educator. One of the first activities I did with SHAPE was "Understanding Your Why." The why was the impetus for delivering the education. I thought back to *Talk Sex* with Sue and my experience with sex education in high-school. This information was not common knowledge. The lack of it was life and death for minoritized identities and seldom was it delivered by people in those communities. "Research suggests that minorities tend to rely heavily on their social networks for health information" (Guzzo & Hayford, 2012). As a community-focused educator, I could corroborate my impact. Serving my community became my first why. I remembered how powerful I felt as a young person in control of my body. I knew pleasure and autonomy were my birthrights. I wanted to gift that revelation to whoever would listen. My last why was based on the speed I integrated topics of human sexuality. I was curious about human sexuality and superb at developing engaging content. Every lesson I received, workshop I gave, and skill I developed released dopamine that I chased to the next experience.

Chasing the dopamine created HonestlyNae, a sexuality education and consultation business for sexuality normalization, explanation, and melanated representation. HonestlyNae exposed the downs of entrepreneurship. I struggled to find spaces that were interested in sex-positive pleasure-focused sexuality education, I planned events no one attended and questioned if I was in the right field. I needed help and guidance. To find a mentor, I hit the conference circuit. I attended as many as possible, sat in on workshops about topics I never heard of, and focused on making sure the educators and professionals I met remembered me. After finding resources, I began to see the ups of entrepreneurship. I collaborated, grew my audiences, and became a household name in the field. Participants would share their life experiences with me after workshops. While some were amenable to my listening and holding space, others wanted help and tools to manifest realities in which they could thrive. To do this, I needed a new set of skills and education.

Sex Therapist

Therapy and education share similar foundations. Both are successful when delivered with energy, attentiveness, authenticity, and confidence. I framed counselling as intensive and individualized education. My clients dictated the lesson plans, and I guided them toward their goals. Counselling is less of a passion than education. It doesn't always trigger a dopamine response, but my skill was needed, and I would serve my community. I named my private practice Manifest Affirm Intention Therapeutic Services because there is magic in words. What we speak we achieve. What we write, we create. Therapy is where that magic can be harnessed and harmonized to produce a reality of the client's creation. My therapeutic approach is humanistic. Humanistic Therapy focuses on the unique lived experience of each individual and emphasizes the capacity for freedom and choice in the process of development and growth. On this basis, humanistic therapies address the personal domain; the interpersonal domain; and clients' reflections on their relationship with self, others, and the wider context of their psychosocial world (Renger & Macaskill, 2021).

My understanding of self came from my personal experiences. Reflecting on impactful moments with a clinical lens helped me push through difficult times, learn from the challenges and celebrate my wins. I wanted to see if this path would help my clients as well. Most of my clients have a minoritized identity, whether it's race, gender, sexuality, or neurodivergence. It is common for this population to focus on adverse emotional reactions and ignore the positive. Sexuality further complicates the issue due to the lack of sex-positive sexuality education accessible to people with minority identities. Many of my clients benefit from education-based sessions early in our relationship. Many have questions about their choices and the outcomes of those choices. Armed with new knowledge, my clients then explore how they can use that information to make decisions aligned with their life goals. Helping my clients understand their active participation in their reality by making choices can remind them of their resilience and capacity. In the following case, I will explore how providing knowledge and supporting choice can help clients uncover and prioritize options aligned with their desires.

Case Study 1: Cesar

In this case study, I explore the impact of language on knowledge of self. With knowledge of self, the client then feels affirmed to make choices that support the expression of his true self.

> *Cesar (he/him) is a 19-year-old Mexican-American heterosexual male. He feels like a "man" but admits to a feminine side that longs to be explored. The man in him also feels conflicted with the kind of man he believes his family and culture expect from him. The Machismo performed in his culture makes him feel like an outsider. "The word machismo has become the social signifier of all that is male chauvinism.. .the epitome of male patriarchal privilege and small-mindedness" (Aida & Mirnal, 2016). He pretends to share their beliefs and mimics their behavior to stay safe from emotional and physical violence. He is worried if his family sees his feminine side, they will assume he is gay. His biggest fear is his Catholic parents disowning him. He does not depend on them for survival resources, but the thought of not interacting with them is heartbreaking. Cesar states he is only romantically and sexually attracted to women. However, he would like to wear "feminine" clothing and not perform stereotypical machismo actions such as anger, aggression, and detachment from his emotions. Cesar presents in therapy to uncover his gender identity and behave authentically. He has no prior knowledge of genders outside of the binary and is open to assistance.*

My hope for this client is to understand gender as a performance and that it has no correlation with sexual orientation. I hope to empower this client to make choices that celebrate his authenticity and give him language to communicate this experience to his parents and community. My goals for this client include the following:

- Expose the client to gender identities that inhabit the masculine and the feminine such as transgender, non-binary, and two-spirit.
- Provide tools to analyze his behaviors and actively make choices that align with his needs.
- Build confidence to invite his parents and community to embrace his whole authentic self

Cesar comes from a traditional religious Latino family. Men in this culture are traditionally protectors, rugged, and stoical. Femininity is seen as weak, not to be aspired to, and shameful if present in men. This is a critical consideration when working therapeutically with him. Cesar understands the rules of Machismo and often chooses to follow that script when he would instead behave differently. I explored with Cesar the moments when he made a different choice than expected. We analyzed what motivated those choices and what the outcomes were. He felt most secure making authentic choices around people with no expectations for him, such as his close friends. After understanding the circumstances of these choices, we put together a safety plan of when he would be free to be authentic and what things he is willing to do to stay safe. Next, we made contact with his feminine energy. We used Gestalt techniques to give the feminine side freedom to speak its needs. Concurrently I recommended YouTube videos, books, podcasts, and movies highlighting people of color with masculine and feminine energy. The more exposure Cesar received, the more language his feminine side developed to communicate its desires. These realizations were new to Cesar and often in conflict with Machismo. In those moments of doubt, I highlighted his resilience and power in choosing what space to be authentic. Cesar relied on his intuition and found comfort in watching other POC celebrate their masculine and feminine genders.

Through our work together, Cesar discovered he was non-binary. I informed him that his sexual orientation and gender identity do not correlate and affirmed his heterosexual identity. Accepting these identities was permission granting. Cesar could lean into whatever energy he chose. Cesar's newfound confidence helped him meet his parents with grace while they grappled with his new identity. He used his journey to understand himself as an anecdote for them. His parent's response further affirmed that all sides of Cesar were essential and deserving to be celebrated.

"Gestalt therapy offers a present-focused, relational approach, central to which is the fundamental belief that the client knows the best way of adjusting to their situation" (Mann, 2021). I used these techniques with Cesar because his culture inundated his behavior. Cesar would need to decide what felt authentic to him and how he wanted to use that information. Increasing his self-awareness and freedom permitted his feminine side to divulge its desires. Discarding those desires felt as if he was rejecting a side of himself. The conjoining of his masculine and feminine unearthed assurance and validity. In this case, we see how awareness, choice, and freedom play a role in the client making decisions based on knowledge and acceptance of self.

Sex Worker

Authenticity is one of the most significant factors in building clientele rapport. My sexuality educator identity and clinician identity developed in my life experiences. They allowed me to connect to my mission, clients, and workshop participants. These identities built businesses, served my community, and fed my passions. I saw no reason my sensual identity should take a back seat when it, too, contributed to my authenticity. My path to sensuality was pleasure derived from my senses. I am particular about how things feel on my skin, how a room smells, and how my food tastes. These particularities were my way of prioritizing pleasure. In my work as an educator, I discovered kink. I researched and practiced the techniques to be an excellent resource. Kink ultimately revealed itself as a multidisciplinary tool.

From my studies, I created a running list of all the archetypes of kink that interested me. I was intrigued by demanding dominance, earning submission, predatory/prey power dynamics, and sensation play. I turned to pop culture for examples of these archetypes and found them all in vampire lore. Vampires are sensual, seductive, dominating, fascinating creatures with a magnetic pull over all others. I knew myself as capable of holding attention and leaving people wanting more. I named this persona Syre and utilized kink as a tool for healing, self-advocacy, and liberation.

I developed skills that matched that of the vampire designed to keep my partners present. Sensation and impact play grants the client the opportunity to inhabit their body. They explore the full capacities of their nervous systems and can use the activity to create and retell narratives derived from their realities. Shibari, also known as Japanese rope bondage, provides restriction and holds the client firmly in the now. Here clients can experience peace in and out of the tension. Tantra is the act of intention. Tantra demands that participants be clear about the outcome and open to the journey. Domination power dynamics are the container that holds my services— the value in choosing to submit honors their yes and no.

Kink is unique in its instant gratification and predictability. Decisions made outside of kink may produce anxiety in waiting for the outcome. To avoid anxiety, people succumb to decision paralysis. Kink participants can witness their choice become action, become gratification, and receive aftercare throughout a scene. There is no need to fear the choice when you can trust you will be supported in its outcome and have the opportunity to modify when necessary.

Case Study 2: Mischief

In this case study, we explore bondage as a tool for body acceptance and how controlling the placement, pattern, and tension of the ropes leads the client to find strength and grace in her body.

> *Mischief (she/her) is a 26-year-old fat Black woman. As a child, she experienced bullying that shaped her self-worth and opinion of her body. Her dislike for her body shows up as an aversion to mirrors, extreme anxiety when shopping for clothes, and disassociation triggered by intimacy. Some of Mischief's idols are Lizzo, Monique, and Gabourey Sidibe. She looks up to them because she aspires to be confident and in charge of her life as they appear to be. Mischief turned to kink to find a way to drown out the negative messages she has of her body and rebuild her confidence. Recently she has been exploring bondage. The thought of being bound feels comforting and relaxing. She is also attracted to the patterns and designs made with the rope. She wants to work with a professional versed in rope, scene negotiation, consent, and aftercare to bring this beautiful and relaxing experience to life.*

My hope for this client is to be an active participant in the placement and tension of the rope. We will focus on areas of the body that hold negativity. Patterns and designs that showcase her body may help her associate it with beauty and joy instead of agony and disgust. The session begins with understanding her wishes and background. I provide education on consent, communication, and an activity overview. I also check on the health and wellness of her body, such as mobility issues and pain. I also note her general attitude toward each section of her body and no touch/yes touch zones.

The rope acted as a dialogue between us. I encouraged her to celebrate her body by creating a unique pattern with the rope. She saw power in the ropes laid on her skin and grace in how they worked with her curves. Eventually, she reflected on how picking clothes were similar to picking how the rope laid on her body. She discovered the power she felt with the ropes could serve her in the store picking clothes. Kink gave her confidence that was transferable into all areas of her life.

The most common question I hear from other professionals is how I navigate dual relationships. I am a multifaceted person that designed a unique path in my career. I wear multiple hats and serve my community in a variety of ways. I have discovered that my clients and workshop attendees find me rooted in the identity that will be of service to them. That identity then becomes the container that supports our relationship. Once a relationship is established, it never wavers. Clinical clients are never allowed to become kink clients and kink clients are never allowed to become clinical. Maintaining this separation creates clear boundaries to be modelled and creates an understanding of the limitations of my skills. I also rely on my mentors and networks for consultation to remain objective and ethical in all my work.

All my personas serve a need I witnessed in my community. I used the energy of passion, pleasure, and dopamine to propel my curiosities. Each persona grew my knowledge and ability arming me with an arsenal of tools influential in many different arenas. Sexuality as a profession is the most exciting, challenging, and freeing experience I have ever had. It is limitless, and there will always be more to learn, experience, teach, and create.

References

Aída Hurtado, & Mrinal Sinha. (2016). *Beyond Machismo: Intersectional Latino Masculinities*. First edition. University of Texas Press. (Accessed December 17, 2022). https://search.ebscohost.com/login.aspx?direct=true&db=nlebk&AN=1139601

Guzzo, K. B., & Hayford, S.R. (2012). Race-Ethnic Differences in Sexual Health Knowledge. *Race Soc Probl.* Dec 1;4(3–4), 158–170. doi: 10.1007/s12552-012-9076-4. Epub 2012 Sep 7. PMID: 23565127; PMCID: PMC3616642

Hatak, I., Chang, M., Harms, R., & Wiklund, J. (2021). ADHD Symptoms, Entrepreneurial Passion, and Entrepreneurial Performance. *Small Business Economics*, 57(4), 1693–1713. https://doi.org/10.1007/s11187-020-00397-x

Mann, D. (2021). *Gestalt Therapy: 100 Key Points & Techniques* (Second ed.). Routledge. https://doi.org/10.4324/9781315158495

Parkes, A., Henderson, M., Wight, D., & Nixon, C. (2011). Is Parenting Associated with Teenagers' Early Sexual Risk-Taking, Autonomy and Relationship with Sexual Partners? *Perspectives on Sexual and Reproductive Health*, 43, 30–40. https://doi.org/10.1363/4303011

Renger, S., & Macaskill, A. (2021). Guided Goal Setting in Therapy Towards being Fully Functioning. *Journal of Contemporary Psychotherapy*, 51(4), 357–364. https://doi.org/10.1007/s10879-021-09505-8

Skuy, P. (1999). *Canadian Pioneers in Family Planning, Journal SOGC*. Elsevier. Available at: https://www.jogc.com/article/S0849-5831(16)30075 1/abstract (Accessed December 17, 2022).

10 REAL Professional Freedom

The Day I Decided to Leave a Group Practice to Start My Own

LaToya Cheathon

Discovery

When I was in middle school, I discovered the career path I was destined to enter—I was going to be a relationship therapist. By this time, I had already spent years being the person who helped mediate conflict in my family and between my friends. I was the go-to person in my group of friends for relationship advice and I had become an advocate for practicing safer-sex amongst my peers. I literally quoted statistics of the risk involved with using various protective methods, and reminded them that nothing protected us 100% from STI's or pregnancy, except abstinence. Yes, this was 12-year-old me who was destined to be a sex and relationship therapist! I knew the first step I needed to take was getting through school by completing a Bachelor's degree in Counseling Psychology, which I did at William Jessup University, and a Master's degree in Counseling Psychology which I completed at National University. Next, in order to get licensed, I needed to obtain 3,000 hours of experience as an Marriage and Family Therapist Intern, as required by the California Board of Behavioral Sciences. In graduate school, I really enjoyed my couples therapy courses, and the singular sex therapy class I took. I knew that I eventually wanted to have my own private practice where I could focus exclusively on helping couples build their best relationship, however, upon completing my graduate program, I found it was very difficult to find a paid internship working with couples that provided enough weekly hours for me to complete all 3,000 hours within two years, which was my personal goal. So, I found myself working at a community mental health agency assisting children and their families where I was able to work full time and complete my hours more quickly. Throughout college and following graduation, I worked various jobs where I learned how to deal with customers, taught preschoolers, provided career counseling to college students, helped foster parents, worked in church counseling centers, emergency departments, crisis lines, substance abuse clinics, and community agencies. By the time I was ten years into my career, I still was not working with couples in private practice like I wanted, and it felt like it was an ever-moving target—always a couple of steps away. I didn't realize it at the time, but every job experience I had

DOI: 10.4324/9781003314660-10

brought me lessons, exposure, and career skills that I would have been avoiding by going straight to private practice. It's important to gain the knowledge and value from each company you work for because you never know how those tools may be needed in the future of your career. Following a cross-country move from Northern California to Atlanta, Georgia, I finally decided it was time to make the transition into private practice, but I felt more comfortable doing so with a safety net of starting part-time while working for a managed care organization and working for someone else's group practice.

So that's what I did, I started with a solo practice owner who was transitioning to a virtual group practice, and she wanted to hire me as her first contracted therapist. I was so excited to work for myself and be able to control how things went for my career, rather than having to conform to the rules and requirements at the large organizations I was used to working for. My hope during that two-year period was to work with someone who was building a group practice so that I could see the steps to building one for myself in the future. I wanted to see how she managed her contractors and employees, how she managed her time, who she hired for support and how she ran the business and financial side of things. I did let the owner of the practice know I was interested in learning more from her, however, she was unable to offer business coaching services to me due to a conflict of interest, which I understood. I also used that time to begin some of the other projects I had always wanted to start, like writing books, carrying out speaking engagements, and building my social media presence.

It's important to note that at the point when I began working for the group practice, it was the year 2020, and the world was beginning to face a global pandemic. There was a lot of uncertainty and fear surrounding what this would mean for business, individual finances, and job security. By the time I left my full-time job in managed care for full time private practice, we were about four months into the pandemic and this was also a time when many people were beginning to reconsider working for others, and starting to open up to the idea of starting their own businesses. This was the beginning of what researcher Ksinan Jiskrova has termed "the Great Resignation," and from my vantage point, many of my therapist friends and colleagues were leaving their full-time jobs and starting their own private practices (2022). During that first year, I had been carrying out speaking engagements, had started a podcast with a colleague, was connecting with other therapists in order to network, and starting various businesses and projects, all from my laptop, because we were all quarantined and afraid of catching Coronavirus. I had started to seriously consider my plan and to wait two more years to start my own practice because finances were a challenge for me, and I wanted to get paid more than the hourly session rate that I had been receiving at the group practice. As a licensed professional, I knew I really didn't *need* to work for anyone, I could just start my own thing and I'd get more income without all of the group practice overheads. I began to feel like I had been holding myself back from leaping in faith because I was struggling with so much imposter syndrome. Some of the negative self-talk I had was "Am I sure I'm ready? Do I really have what it takes? Am I organized enough? Am I smart enough? Can I even be successful on my own?" I went back and forth with myself on these questions for several months, talking myself into and out of it repeatedly, thinking the timing wasn't right, that I needed to be better equipped, or that there really was no rush to run off by myself. However, after much consideration, and with little preparation, I handed in my notice about six months earlier than the two years I had planned, told myself to "do it scared," and launched into my own private practice, Happily Attached Sex and Relationship Therapy! So, here I am—two years into full-time private practice, and one year out on my own, and I want to share some of the insight on the lessons I've learned post "leap," that I wish I had considered before making the move, because as most of us know, hindsight tends to be clearer.

Getting Started

When getting started as a new practice owner, it's so important to begin by learning the business side of it all. This is an area that most mental health graduate school programs and sex therapy school programs do not teach their students, which sets many future practice owners up for a rocky start. Starting this type of business is the same as it would be for any other type of business—by first identifying the mission and vision for the business and developing a business plan. This starts the process of setting your business apart from other businesses with a unique core identity. In research from Ingenhoff and Fuhrer, a business' mission statement is a sentence describing the company's function, what sets them apart from competitors, and the goals and philosophies of the business (Ingenhoff & Fuhrer, 2010). According to Entreprenuer.com, a mission statement should explain what the business has to offer, who the business serves, and how they help the customers (*Mission Statement – Entrepreneur Small Business Encyclopedia*, 2022). For me, my business is a therapy practice that specializes in helping People of Color improve their relationships, and address any sex-related challenges using attachment-based therapy techniques. My mission statement is "Happily Attached Sex and Relationship Therapy is a mental health and wellness practice focused on helping Couples from marginalized backgrounds improve the intimacy, connection and communication within their relationships."

According to Peek from *Business News Daily*, a company's vision should communicate the ideal long-term business goals, and it should reflect your view of the world and your business's place in it. (Peek, 2022) I had to ask myself what I wanted my business to look like over time. Since my business is an extension of me and my values and beliefs, this should be reflected in my vision statement. My passion is helping couples thrive in relationships by gaining a better understanding of their individual needs and desires, and learning tools to assist in communicating those needs and desires to those around them. Additionally, I feel like there are not enough resources out there for couples therapists to have mentoring and supervision provided by therapists who specialize in working with couples. My vision statement is "Happily Attached will become the go-to couples therapy practice, providing services to couples from marginalized communities in various states across the United States, and healing families by starting with strengthening the relationship between the couples." Some of my business' projected outcomes include hiring both pre-licensed and fully licensed couples therapists from across America to see clients, hiring clinical supervisors to provide supervision for the pre-licensed clinicians, and growing the business to having at least ten employees within the first five years.

To identify the goals for my business, it was important to start with creating a business plan, which the US Small Business Administration describes as "a roadmap for structuring, running and growing the business." (https://www.sba.gov/business-guide) Beginning with the end in mind, it is important to identify the long-term goals for the business and have a rough idea of the strategies to get there. Developing a plan for my business was a step that I did, which is "what" I wanted it to look like, however, I didn't spend enough time looking at the "how" I would get there. For example, I knew I wanted to eventually develop my solo practice into a group practice by adding clinicians and providing training and supervision to therapists in the field. However, I was unaware that setting this up was something that needed more time than I was expecting it to take, and that each step would build upon the last and wouldn't be done simultaneously. I wish I had taken the time before I left the group practice to really flush out the steps I needed to take to get certified as a supervisor, and to become more familiar with things like employment laws in my state and financial planning within business.

Building up my knowledge on marketing became the next challenge for me when I started my business. What I learned through attending workshops and training on this topic was that I had to really get into the minds of my ideal clients and consider their pain points. Merriam-Webster defines a "pain point" as "a persistent or recurring problem (as with a product or service) that frequently inconveniences or annoys customers" (*Pain Point*, n.d.). So, I had to research to learn more about my ideal clients—what issues or concerns did they feel they dealt with repeatedly in their relationships? What kind of negative thoughts did they have about their relationships? How may they have sought to remedy this in the past, and in what ways have their previous support resources not met their needs? Many business owners may conduct online research or poll people they know to gather this information. The most important part is to really try to put yourself in the shoes of the population you want to serve, in order to identify what they really want, which could be different than what they are asking for. For example, a client may come to me and say that they want to stop fighting so much with their partner. What they may actually be asking for are ways to effectively communicate their needs to their partner in a way that makes them feel empowered, valued and heard. The client may not realize there is a way to improve the dynamics in their communication with their partner so that the two may be able to have productive conversations, so maybe they feel like they just want to stop the fighting. However, if I can come from their perspective, I may be able to add wording to my website that lets them know, for example "I help couples build skills to address even their most challenging communication issues to resolve their conflicts and walk away from the conversations feeling heard and more connected with their partner." This type of a description is more likely to grab the reader's attention and create hope that I may be the person who can finally help them because my words are speaking to their exact pain points. Really spending a considerable amount of time developing these types of descriptions was not something I prioritized in the beginning because I didn't realize how important it actually was. Had I taken the time to really get into the minds of my ideal client beforehand, I may have had more initial success with attracting clients who I truly wanted to work with. Instead, I took on whatever couples I could get, for example, taking on many insurance-based clients, because it produced a steady stream of referrals, rather than taking the time to improve my marketing to attract my ideal clients who would pay out of pocket. I have always envisioned keeping my practice as only private pay for a few reasons. The first is that many insurance companies do not cover couples therapy. Second, the rate the insurance companies pay is a lot less than the fee I charge for therapy sessions. Another reason is that I do not want to deal with the hassle of filing claims, and waiting for insurance companies to send out payment for my client's sessions. Finally, I've observed that people are more invested in therapy when it is something they are paying for out of pocket, rather than just paying a copayment for their services.

Since my business is focused on servicing People of Color, that is reflected in the people on the images I use on my website, and even on my logo and email signature, I have the words "specializing in Couples of Color." This is to let my ideal clients, who are people from historically marginalized communities, know that Happily Attached is a place they are welcomed, and it is for them, not just a generic place for everyone. Research shows that Black clients in particular strongly prefer working with a Black therapist, according to Goode-Cross and Grim (2014). Based on what I have heard from clients since beginning my practice, People of Color in general want to meet with another Person of Color, even if they are not from the same racial background. My clients have shared that they specifically sought me out as a therapist because they were looking for a therapist who was a Black woman, or a Person of Color. A lot of people may hesitate to niche down and advertise to a specific demographic because they don't want to shut others out. This was a mild concern for me, as well. However, through the various trainings I did on building a business, I was reminded of a couple of things: 1) I am not here to serve everyone, I am here to serve *some* people and 2) those who want to work with me, will come to me, even if they are not part of the demographic I am advertising to. I've worked with many couples who do not identify as People of Color who came to me for therapy, and were not dissuaded from contacting me because of my advertised mission. I work with couples who are from all backgrounds, however, in my messaging, I made sure to speak directly to those I created my business to help. I choose to believe that clients who are meant to work with me will come to me, and anyone who does not become my client was not meant to work with me, and they will hopefully find their way to a therapist who is a better fit for their needs.

In addition, as part of my business development, I didn't know how the addition of the word "sex" into my company's name, and having it as one of the primary focuses of my business, would affect things since the word "sex" has such a stigma in American society. As I began adding content to my social media, I initially wanted to help reduce that stigma by just using the word "sex" as needed, figuring that people not talking about it is a large part of the problem, and it just perpetuates the issue. However, my social media manager came to me one day to share that she noticed that the content with images and titles using the word "sex" had been viewed by fewer people due to the social media algorithm blocking many from see-ing the posts. She suggested we instead try coding the word, as many other sex education and sex therapy accounts on social media had been doing, with terms like "s3x" or "s*x." This appeared to improve the overall reach of my posts. By looking at the engagement and reach on my social media pages in the "Insights" section of my account, we were also able to see that there is a significantly higher level of interest and engagement in posts that talk about sex-related concerns, over the other types of content I post about relationships in general. Since sex is a taboo topic that many strug-gle with, but have shame and discomfort in discussing with anyone else (sometimes even with their partner), utilizing social media as a resource to normalize their concerns, and provide some education and point them to sex-positive resources has proven to be appreciated and needed. This has been increasing my overall business influence and professional credibility in the online world.

As a result of directing my focus on improving my social media presence and becoming a source of helpful information, I have received numerous emails and messages on social media inviting me to assist in the advertise-ment of various products, invitations to speak at conferences and on pod-casts, received free gifts and products, and offered many opportunities to collaborate with other professionals in different fields. These have proven to be an additional source of income, as well as exposure to more potential contracts and roles. I even created a networking group for Therapists of Color in my city, and have made many connections and have received a lot of referrals through them via word-of-mouth. Utilizing networking oppor-tunities to connect with other professionals, and leveraging my expertise to create additional income has been something else I learned to do in my first year on my own. As an entrepreneur, I realized having multiple streams of income can be very helpful during slow times in my business or to assist in reaching my financial goals. One thing that I considered several times in the first year when things got slow, was whether it made more sense to go back into the workforce and get a part time job working for someone else. Each time I had to really evaluate why I was looking into that option, and I learned it had a lot to do with my own personal financial fears, limited mindset and the feelings of uncertainty related to my first year in business. Where you place your focus, that's where the money will flow, so I had to learn not to get distracted by other jobs, trying to take an easier way out, because in the long run, my goals were to pour back into my own business, rather than trying to speed up the process of increasing my income by pouring into someone else's business. Each business owner will have to make the best decision for him/herself, but the main thing I wanted to point out was that money mindset issues will likely be revealed during the first year of a new business, so getting ahead of that and having a better understanding of your beliefs about money can be a good way to gain clarity and direction for use during difficult times.

This was another area that has been a steep learning curve for me—getting my business finances in order. Since I did not have a background in finances, and since graduate school did not prepare me to be a business owner, I walked into this business with limited knowledge on how to start and manage a small business financially. Some resources that were helpful for me have been to join various Facebook groups focused on financial literacy and mindset for mental health providers in private practice, hiring a bookkeeper and tax accountant, and reading highly recommended books like Profit First and others to better understand this part. Once I had a better understanding of how my money flowed in and out of my business, I was able to identify whom I could hire to assist me in the areas of my business that I did not have expertise in, or areas I simply did not want to handle myself. It's important as a business owner to know your limitations and set boundaries around your time and energy. According to Forbes.com, there are four types of scenarios a business owner will have—no income, low-income, high-income, and legacy building. They recommend delegating all tasks that are no income or low-income to make more time for the high-income and legacy building tasks (Djavid, 2022). Investing in the right kind of help, can make the flow of the business run so much more smoothly. Creating systems and structures can lead to greater productivity and effectiveness in a business from the start, so hiring experts in the areas of setting up these systems can save a lot of time, energy, and headache for the business owner.

When I made the move from working at a group practice into my own solo practice, it was quite a journey for me. I waited longer than I needed to because I was holding myself back, feeling like an imposter, and not realizing that I already had what it took to be successful. I participated in a lot of training, and at times I believe I even got stuck in learning mode, as a procrastination tactic to avoid moving forward into my greatness. I had to learn that at a certain point, it's time to stop learning and start doing, with authority, even when in doubt. However, the key is in both the preparation before the leap, and a business owner's ability to not lose focus early on in the midst of trials. Some businesses really struggle in the first few years, so having a business coach or mentor can be helpful for the new business owner to check in with to see if it would be wise to continue with their business as it is, or if they may need to make some shifts in their business model in order to stay afloat. Learning ways to work smarter, not harder, remaining focused on long-term career goals, understanding the business and financial side of entrepreneurship, leveraging social media influence, networking, and delegating as needed were the most important pillars of my success in my first year of business. It is important to remember that the freedom of entrepreneurship comes at a price, as with more freedom comes more responsibility, and less external accountability. This process has required me to set boundaries, put in many long hours, make decisions all on my own, and be fully responsible for the outcomes. For me, it was well worth it. I was stretched so much in areas I didn't even realize I needed growth in and I became exactly who I was meant to be. And I am continuing to learn and flourish more each day. I am so glad that I didn't let fear hold me back and that I chose to take the leap from working for others, into owning my own successful business, and having *REAL professional freedom*!

Questions for Reflection

1. How have your various jobs prepared you for your future as a business owner and expert in your field?
2. What structures and systems do you want to have set up that your future-self will thank you for? How can you set yourself up to be ready so you don't have to get ready?
3. How do you feel about using social media to grow our business and help you reach a larger audience? What do you think people see when pulling up your business online?
4. How can you set yourself up for success by mentally preparing for what will be required as a business owner? How do you know if hiring a business coach would be helpful for you?
5. Who are some people you know in business that you can be more intentional about networking with? Remember, they don't have to be in your field—diversify your connections!

References

Djavid, N. (2022, January 19). *Business Owners: Determine Your Essential Tasks and Delegate The Rest.* Forbes. https://www.forbes.com/sites/forbesbusinessc ouncil/2022/01/19/business-owners-determine-your-essential-tasks-and-delegate -the-rest/?sh=740e29f72daf

Goode-Cross, D. T., & Grim, K. A. (2014). An Unspoken Level of Comfort. *Journal of Black Psychology*, *42*(1), 29–53. https://doi.org/10.1177/0095798414552103

Ingenhoff, D., & Fuhrer, T. (2010). Positioning and differentiation by using brand personality attributes. *Corporate Communications: An International Journal*, *15*(1), 83–101. https://doi.org/10.1108/13563281011016859

Ksinan Jiskrova, G. (2022). Impact of COVID-19 pandemic on the workforce: from psychological distress to the Great Resignation. *Journal of Epidemiology and Community Health*, *76*(6), 525–526. https://doi.org/10.1136/jech-2022-218826

Mission Statement – Entrepreneur Small Business Encyclopedia. (2022, December 21). Entrepreneur. https://www.entrepreneur.com/encyclopedia/mission-statement

Pain Point. (n.d.). The Merriam-Webster.com Dictionary. https://www.merriam -webster.com/dictionary/pain%20point

Peek, S. (2022, November 22). *What Is a Vision Statement?* Business News Daily. https://www.businessnewsdaily.com/3882-vision-statement.html

US Small Business Administration. (2022). https://www.sba.gov/business-guide/plan -your-business/write-your-business-plan

11 Finding Your Niche

The Importance of Specialization and Branding

Quantas L. Ginn

Helping clients embrace and flourish in their sexuality is a task well served by sex therapists the world over. These clinicians address a wide spectrum of sexual concerns client bring into the therapy room. Sex therapy is a unique field because of the "knowledge about human sexuality and sexology that practitioners must acquire during the training process" (Kleinplatz, 2009). It is a practice which examines as Levine (2009) puts it, "the interaction of the past and present, the individual and the partner, the body and the culture." Sex therapy itself is a niche within the field of psychotherapy. But even within the world of sex therapy there are niches (aka specializations) which clinicians can lean into.

Arguably, the most effective sex therapists operate within a specialization catered to certain populations. A specialist, as opposed to a generalist, has the opportunity to provide deeper, more knowledgeable support. Operating as a "jack of all trades" has the potential to lead to burnout and/or disinterest within the clinician as well as poor client outcomes. In this chapter we will explore why it is important for sex therapists to know their niche, how to find their niche, and then how to effectively reach their niche.

What is a Niche?

Before we discuss how to find our niche, it is necessary to define what is a niche. A niche is an area of focus or specialization within a larger context. Sex therapy itself is a niche within the field of psychotherapy. And within sex therapy there are a variety of issues to focus upon. These can include arousal disorder, erectile dysfunction, perinatal issues, asexuality, pelvic floor pain, out of control sexual behavior (OCSB)/ "sex addiction," ethical nonmonogamy, disabled folks, trans folks, sex and aging, kink, sexual trauma, religious sexual shame, sex work, and BDSM. Additionally, there are some sex therapists specifically trained to work with sex offenders or minor-attracted individuals. Another helpful approach could be to categorize the needs client present around male bodies, female bodies, queer bodies, trans bodies, older bodies, and/or disabled bodies. Going forward, the terms niche and specialization will be utilized interchangeably.

DOI: 10.4324/9781003314660-11

Why Is a Niche Important?

The importance of having your niche is to the benefit of your clients as well as to you, the clinician. It is equally important for both parties involved. For clinicians, it is imperative we know our strengths, passions, and limitations. We are not a good fit for every client. We do not, and cannot, know everything. As the old saying goes, "…a jack of all trades but a master of none." It is not possible to serve all folks well. Along the way someone or something suffers. The one who suffers may be the clinician themselves in the form of professional burnout (i.e., disinterest, cynicism, or exhaustion). In this space, providing therapy could feel like an obligation or a burden instead of an energizing passion. Or your clients who need a clinician with a special set of skills to address their needs. In an effort to make yourself and your practice more sustainable serving your ideal client is a must.

Essentially, the more passionate and knowledgeable we are in with their particular needs the more effective we can be in moving them toward their sexual wellness goals. Granted, as previously mentioned, sex therapy itself is a niche within the larger field of psychotherapy, there are certain issues which may be better served with a therapist with a particular set of skills. These could include such issues as pelvic floor pain, polyamory, out of control sexual behavior (OCSB), trans care, or sex work.

There are, however, differing opinions regarding sex therapists having a niche. A few colleagues whom I discussed this topic felt that the work of the sex therapist is to help their clients with all their sexual wellness needs. One sexuality educator emphatically disagreed with having a niche and emphasized the need to take a holistic approach (Fredrick Zal, 2022). They went on to say,

> I have always been a "generalist", as people do not exist in niches. People are complex, and I feel that we as professionals need to meet people where they are. I do not want to shoehorn someone into a predefined niche, especially if that was formed for capitalistic marketing reasons.

Another colleague also highlighted this fact: many times, our clients have co-occurring issues which tie into other work we may be addressing (Brittany Steffen, 2022). In these instances, breaking the therapeutic relationship could be detrimental to the client's progress. Steffen goes on to describe her experience with therapists referring out when it was not in the best interest of the client:

> …[the] therapist said, "I don't work with that issue" and referred the client out. I feel like this is discrimination—when we have a client, we constantly see new issues pop up that we're not super familiar with, and we are required to educate ourselves so we can continue to support our

clients. When a therapist refers out a client, research tells us that most of the time, that client never follows through with finding additional treatment. That leaves this already underserved and marginalized population without care and appropriate mental health treatment, in a world where they may face daily discrimination, as well as housing and job insecurity, among other things. The pain and devastation that those clients experienced when their therapists broke off their therapeutic relationship with them, after they talked about gender identity, was awful to witness.

These points illustrate an important point. Specialization should not be the main focal point if client care suffers. Our aim as sex therapists is to provide care for our clients and the issues they present. To this end, it is imperative that we continue to be humble, curious, and ever learning to serve the clients in front of us well. Additionally, as we evolve as clinicians, our niches will naturally evolve and expand. This would be expected. The way forward between the specialist vs. generalist approach could be leaning into a specialty but continually increasing our skill set to systemically address the myriad of issues a client may present.

Finding Your Niche

Now that we have discussed the importance of having a niche, now it is time to discuss how we each can find the specialit(ies) in which we lean. To discover one's niche there are several methods to utilize. The process involves by first looking at oneself through self-reflection, possibly soliciting feedback from family, friends, and colleagues and then observing one's surroundings (i.e., unfulfilled client needs, local available offerings, etc.).

Drawing from the fundamentals of business marketing, the concept of the 5 P's is a helpful starting point when thinking of finding your niche. The 5 P's of marketing include product, price, promotion, place, and people (Canella, 2015). Product is defined as the good or service being offered in the marketplace. In the field of sex therapy, *you*, the clinician, are the product. Your skills, knowledge, empathy, curiosity, and personality are what clients are procuring. With an understanding of you being the product, the process of self-reflection can help you understand what you have and want to offer.

Self-Reflection

Self-reflection is a fruitful way to gain insight into your passions and curiosities. To home into these passions one useful exercise is as followed:

- *Reflect upon the sessions you have had with clients in which you felt the most refreshed and energized afterwards.*

This can illuminate your own gravitational pull. Working within your passions can bring about an attitude of "I get to…" instead of "I have to…"

Following your curiosities has a way of leading you to your niche. Think about *which trainings do you continually find yourself drawn? What topics do you continually ponder over? What readings left you wanting more? What conversations piqued your curiosity?* As one colleague described to me, they followed their curiosities and the opportunities came (Fredrick Zal, 2022).

Another exercise to include in your self-reflection would be uncovering your *"why."* *Why did you decide to become a sex therapist? What did you envision you doing to help clients achieve their sexual wellness?* It could be as simple as finishing this sentence: *"I am a sex therapist because…."* One Black colleague stated his "why" by simply stating his desire to help "people who look like me" (Greg Dawson II, 2022).

To further reveal your "why," reflect upon your own sexual wellness journey. Out of our own pain or frustrations we can remember why we decided to become a sex therapist. Out of our own confusion or pain, we can identify who we want to be for our clients. Our joys and pleasures as well as our pain and struggles have helped shaped who we are and who we are becoming. This is a part of who is showing up in the therapy room for clients. This approach is gleaning insights from the past.

An approach of starting from the future and working backwards is asking yourself the question: *What do I want my legacy to be as a sex therapist?* And be specific. A phrasing such as, "At the end of my career, I want to be known as a sex therapist who helped black femmes embrace, own, and flourish in their sexual expression and enjoyment."

Feedback from Others

Sometimes we need feedback from those closest to us to identify who we are. *Who would your friends and family say that you are?* Are you the one who seeks to care the forgotten, the marginalized? Are you the one who seeks to care for the traumatized and hurting? Are you the one who has always been drawn to the shamed and outcasts of society? As we know, within the field of sex therapy there are various populations who have felt this way about themselves, and it is interrupting their journey to sexual wellness. Professional colleagues provide helpful sources of information too. *Whom do you find yourself regularly associating? What do they see in you? Which colleagues do you find yourself drawn to?*

Unfulfilled Client Needs

I found this niche as it is a mirror of who I am. I found in my own journey, these identities were not well represented, researched, nor written about which felt lonely and isolating. A defining moment for me was searching for a therapist of color (black), who knew sex therapy, and was queer and really coming up empty. I knew at that moment that I needed to step up as a therapist. I could not be the only one looking for someone like me.

(Anthony Pennant, 2022)

Another colleague kept seeing gaps in what was offered in the community from what clients were presenting with and what they were hearing from colleagues (Mia Fine, 2022).

Discovering Along the Way

"Sometimes the work finds you by happenstance" (Nicole Wilson, 2022). Along our journey we will naturally find our ideal clients and our ideal clients will find us. Or sometimes clients find you first and then you find your calling (Brittany Steffen, 2022). A type of Law of Attraction at work.

Reaching your niche

Once you have found the specializations in which you want to focus, the next step is to reach your ideal client. Stepping into the mind of your clients will inform how to best connect. In the field of marketing this is called psychographics. Borrowing from our field of psychology, marketing professionals examine the intersection of demographics and psychological factors within their target market (Samuel, 2016). The list below details some of the information which could help identify the ways in which to engage potential clients:

Psychographic Profile Information

Age	Income
Race	Education level
Sex	Spiritual practice
Gender	Current living situation
Relationship status	Hobbies
Number of children	Presenting issues (as defined by them)
Types of media consumption	

Detailing this information can help you envision who are your ideal clients. Below are some examples of potential ideal clients. The first could be for a sex therapist in a medium-sized Midwest city in the United States who wants to help their clients thrive in their sexuality.

Ideal Client #1: "Jan"

Jan is a married middle-aged white woman with two teenagers at home. She is comfortably middle class and has stable employment as a middle-school teacher. Jan considers herself a Christian but does not regularly practice her faith. Jan is somewhat tech savvy: she regularly uses popular social media sites and is proficient at finding information online. In her free time, she likes to spend time outdoors and gardening. When it comes to her sexuality, Jan feels unfulfilled and dissatisfied. She knows there is more she could be experiencing but she does not know how to get there or where to turn.

This next profile could be for a sex therapist who wants to provide a space for marginalized queer Black folk in large city in the southeastern United States.

Ideal Client #2: "Trevor"

Trevor is a late twenty-something Black man who identifies as pansexual. He is working class and works at a national retail store. Trevor grew up in a conservative religious home where his effeminate presentation was not welcomed and overtly discouraged. Trevor is tech-savvy and heavily uses the latest apps and social media networks. He finds community online and struggles to find community locally. When it comes to his sexuality, Trevor struggles with self-acceptance and feeling marginalized. He wants to fully live out who he is and find long-term love.

Now what do we do with this knowledge to better reach our clients? How did this knowledge affect our marketing efforts? This information should be used in the messaging we place on our practice websites, online directories, etc. to speak to our ideal client's passions, hopes, dreams, and pain points. Envisioning your ideal client will inform which imagery and photographs to use. Ideally choosing images that either reflect the clients themselves or imagery in which they can identify.

Your publicity and promotions plans will be impacted by this information as well. (Publicity is free and comes in the forms of such things as press coverage, speaking engagements, and article contributions. Promotions are paid opportunities such as Google Ads, Facebook Ads, and online directories.) Where are your clients spending their time, virtually and in real life? Are they on the latest social media network? Are they attending groups in person? This determines where they will find and hear your message.

Hall and Binik (2020) note the trend in which sex therapy is taking on a more interdisciplinary approach. Nowadays many sex therapists find themselves collaborating with urologists, pelvic floor therapists, and gynecologists

(Hall & Binik, 2020). These could be rich referral sources as well. Trevor, the ideal client previously mentioned, may be discussing his struggles with a local support group for queer Black folks. Collaborating with groups like these through providing workshops or blog posts could prove to be a useful source of referrals.

Conclusion

As we clinicians seek to help our clients thrive in their sexuality, striving to master a niche is an important path to serving our clients well. This can provide an opportunity to provide thorough, knowledgeable support. Specializing also has a way of decreasing the chance of burnout and/or poor client outcomes.

Hopefully this text has illuminated the importance of sex therapists to knowing their niche, finding their niche, and a way forward to effectively reach their niche.

Questions for Reflection

As we reflect upon finding our niche(s), the questions below can help us better explore the path ahead:

1. Why did I become a sex therapist?
2. What impact do I want to have?
3. Who are "my people?"
4. How do I better serve my ideal clients?
5. Am I cognizant of how I am evolving as a sex therapist?

References

Canella, M. (2015). *Session 3: Marketing. University of Vermont Farmer Training Program* [PowerPoint slides]. Retrieved from https://blog.uvm.edu/farmvia/files /2015/07/Session-3-Marketing-2015.pdf

Dawson II, G. (2022, April). Sex Therapist. Personal communication [phone interview].

Fine, M. (2022, May–June). Sex Therapist. Personal communication [phone interview and email].

Hall, K. S. K., & Binik, Y. M. (2020). *Principles and practice of sex therapy.* pp. 512.

Kleinplatz, P. (2009). Consumer protection is the major purpose of sex therapy certification. *Archives of Sexual Behavior, 38:* 1031–1032 DOI 10.1007/ s10508-009-9473-y

In J. C. Norcross & M. R. Goldfried (Eds.), *Handbook of psychotherapy integration* (pp. 94–129). New York: Basic Books.

Levine, S. B. (2009). I am not a sex therapist! *Archives of Sexual Behavior, 38*: 1033–1034 DOI 10.1007/s10508-009-9474-x

Pennant, A. (2022, May). Sex Therapist. Personal communication [E-mail].

Samuel, A. (2016, March 11). Psychographics are just as important for marketers as demographics. *Harvard Business Review*. https://hbr.org/2016/03/psychographics -are-just-as-important-for-marketers-as-demographics

Steffen, B. (2022, May–June). Sex Therapist. Personal communication [E-mail].

Wilson, N. (2022, April). Personal communication [E-mail].

Zal, F. (2022, May). Sexuality Educator. Personal communication [E-mail].

12 The Business of Sex Coaching

13 Steps to Career Success as a Sexological Entrepreneur

Patti Britton and Sarah Martin

Introduction

Sexology is an interdisciplinary discipline that encompasses all profession-als within the field, such as sexuality educators, sex therapists, sexuality counselors, sex coaches, sex researchers, and medical or mental health pro-fessionals who touch on aspects of sexual wellness in their unique areas of care and expertise. A plethora of education and training opportunities exist that elevate the knowledge and clinical skills level of sexologists. Just look at the Continuing Education listings at AASECT[1] or the content scope at any sexology conference, such as the Society for the Scientific Study of Sexuality (SSSS),[2] World Congresses of the World Association for Sexual Health (WAS),[3] or specialty sexuality educational events. One missing ingredient, however, in almost all sexuality-related training programs is a thorough, robust, comprehensive, and complete educational track in business success. One has only to scan the graduate programs in psychology, medical schools, or AASECT or WAS type of offerings to see that how to succeed in busi-ness, as a sexological entrepreneur, is the hidden longing and unmet need of most practicing or aspiring clinicians. To answer that call, along came Sex Coach U.

The history of Sex Coach U began in 2010, when Britton and her then life and business partner Robert Dunlap (deceased in 2017), founded the online training and certification program known as Sex Coach U. Britton and Dunlap were accomplished and highly respected clinical sexologists with unique backgrounds as entrepreneurs, all of which informed the crea-tion and ongoing development of a specialized, cutting-edge, pioneering entity. Since that time other coaching programs have surfaced offering dif-ferent methodologies for the training of sex coaches. Sex coaching as a new profession, little known to educators or clinicians before, was created by its pioneer, Britton, also the author of the first (and to date the only) text-book on sex coaching, *The Art of Sex Coaching: Expanding Your Practice* (Norton, 2005). The first iteration of Sex Coach U was built around the combination of the "what" of sexology and the "how" of coaching. The

DOI: 10.4324/9781003314660-12

curriculum also contained a taste of business education, such as forming a vision for your business, simple one-year business plans, tasks for following your numbers, creating a disaster recovery plan for future emergencies, and a smattering of basics that served to awaken preparedness for the entrepreneurial acumen needed among its students. After nine years of graduating hundreds of competent and qualified Certified Sex Coaches™ from the program, it became clear that, although these grads were knowledgeable and well prepared to serve the *clinical* concerns of their clients, few were thriving financially.

To address this gap in entrepreneurial acumen and skills, a new vision emerged and the Business of Sex Coaching (BOSC) program[4] was created by the two authors, Britton and Martin, in 2019. Their years of experience and extensive business training were perfectly tailored to address the specific needs of sex coaches (and applicable for other sexuality professionals) for building a thriving, sustainable private practice that could flourish. The current curricular structure at Sex Coach U is a triadic model: Sexology, Coaching, and Business form the three prongs of the training a student experiences through a program that can take up to 800 hours to complete. Currently, over 200+ graduates represent the scope of influence Sex Coach U has in over 75 countries around the globe. The Sex Coach U Business of Sex Coaching component is in vibrant motion to inform, train, and empower the current students in this groundbreaking program.

This chapter covers the vision and content of BOSC. It offers a practical guide for the reader to gain an overview of what any independent sexuality professional, especially one who identifies as an entrepreneur, must know and be able to do to thrive in business. The chapter provides a look at the full journey a BOSC student takes, including the outcome expectations that are embedded in the journey.

The Business of Sex Coaching Program

The Business of Sex Coaching program guides students to develop both an Inner Game and Outer Game to create a well-rounded approach to building a thriving private practice. Inner Game is the foundation of entrepreneurial wellness, including Extreme Self-Care, Money Mindset, and Prosperity Consciousness. Outer Game includes strategic planning and practical guidelines with steps toward effective implementation. BOSC is a powerful container for students to stretch, grow, and thrive on this profound personal and professional journey. In the BOSC program, participants confront old wounds around what they deserve, learn to make love to their money, find abundance for their lives, and master the 13 steps involved in building a successful sex coaching business that endures.

The 13 Steps to Sexuality Business Mastery

1. Make extreme self-care a daily habit to support you through the entrepreneurial journey. Cultivate courage, self-belief, and self-worth as you manage your time, energies, and vision for your future.
2. Tune your money mindset to prosperity consciousness for life and business. Find inspiration, daily habits, and make a practice of noticing the abundance all around you.
3. Set up your mind, emotions, body, energy, spirit, and working space for money attraction.
4. Establish money management habits and engage in a positive relationship with your money.
5. Create business planning strategies that prioritize what's important to you and your business. Use your strategies to make better decisions.
6. Discover your ideal client and get to know and understand the essence of your ideal client, including their pains, fears, hopes, dreams, and the language used to describe them.
7. From the start, create products that serve your clients. Set up pricing that permits you to thrive.
8. Create and expand educational products that allow you to serve many people at once. Maximize your ability to productize all you have to offer.
9. Develop your ability to speak confidently and succinctly to anyone about what you do as a professional.
10. Cultivate a web presence that spreads your message and reaches your ideal client.
11. Set up systems for consistency in marketing and launching your products and services. Know how to attract and use effective steps for filling your funnel.
12. Sell from a mindset of "service" and systematize the process of welcoming new clients.
13. Reinvest in your business for growth and scaling. Be ready to outsource tasks to software and people for your business success.

Inner Game and Entrepreneurial Wellness

As a sexuality professional, nine times out of ten, you are your business. That's why it's vital that your work stems from a stable, confident core. Your Inner Game is the mindset that allows you to show up fully in your business with grace, strength, and resilience. It is the foundation for your success and longevity in the field of sexuality. Inner Game work is an ongoing deep dive inside you. It involves all of your thoughts, feelings, and attitudes. Inner Game means working with your blockages, prejudices, and -isms. On this journey of growth as a business owner, you will meet both the scared parts of you and the excited parts of you.

Cultivating Inner Game is an invitation to befriend your demons. It may come as a surprise that your demons will come up in the process of building a private practice. Many new entrepreneurs don't fully understand just how much personal development and self-confrontation is required to get a business off the ground. When you first hear the critical voice of your self-doubt, it's easy to stop in your tracks. Inner Game means learning to embrace those demons, knowing how to live with your gremlins (e.g., insecurities, anxieties, and fears), and discovering how to catch all of those fear-based voices and turn them into positive operating systems.

The work of Inner Game is also a cyclical process of continually building capacity for success. For you, like for many entrepreneurs, stumbling upon your fears related to success can be a revelation. Who doesn't want to be successful, after all? Why wouldn't you want to be well-known, in-demand, and highly compensated? But until you have stretched your capacity to comfortably hold abundance, it will continue to elude you. While Inner Game work must come first as an integral part of the foundations of your business, it is never done. It is a journey you will be on every day for the rest of your business, and for the rest of your life.

Extreme Self-Care

Inner Game is the foundation of your business, and extreme self-care is the foundation of Inner Game. In order to create, launch, and run your own sex coaching business, you have to become an expert at self-care, which means that you need to be selfish. Yes, selfish! Essentially, self-care means taking care of number one—that's you—at all times. You must come first. You cannot take care of others, whether it's your family, coworkers, clients, or students, unless and until you have taken care of yourself. You have to put on your own oxygen mask before you can help others. What's more, your self-care serves as a role model for the empowerment of your clients.

Try Out These 7 Sample Actions for Extreme Self-Care

- Meditate as often or regularly as you can. Even two minutes can be enough to reset you for smooth sailing throughout your day.
- Use positive affirmations. We now know from neuroscience that affirmations work. What you tell yourself matters. So be nice to yourself.

- Take real time off where you spend some time off grid taking a break from technology and the endless devices you interact with every day.
- Take time alone to just be and stoke the fire of your own self connection.
- Have an active sense of humor. Laughter really does heal. Watch funny shows or go to a standup comedy act.
- Exercise, whether it's a workout in a gym, a yoga class, riding a horse, bike riding, anything that's physically challenging will open up oxygen flow, release feel good hormones, and energize you.
- Set real, firm, and ongoing healthy boundaries. Create boundaries to protect your mental, emotional, physical, spiritual, and energetic self.

For effective, sustaining self-care, you must conserve and ruthlessly protect your most valuable resource as an entrepreneur: your energy. You need to address where people, thoughts, things, or the niggling undone parts of your life or business are stealing your energy. How will you notice and let go of whatever is draining you and move toward powering yourself up with energy gaining replacements? Spend time at the beginning or end of every work week taking stock of your current Energy Drainers, like doom scrolling, that family member who calls you every day to complain, or the one client who texts you out of hours, and making a plan to convert them into Energy Gainers, like reading a paper book, spending time with people who light you up, and setting clear boundaries with your clients. Notice where your life and your business are in flow and balance and where they are not. This concept is derived from the tenets of life coaching.[5] Make this a habit. The more you practice noticing Energy Drainers and replacing them with Energy Gainers, the easier it will become.

You can further strengthen your self-care practice by using the power of ritual. If ritual as a word turns you off or pushes you away, think of ritual like a shortcut for habit formation. Love it or hate it, ritual allows you to tap into powerful parts of the human brain that respond to routine and intentional practice. For example, a daily ritual can mark your transition into the work day. Having that conscious transition from one state to another can be especially helpful if you work from home. Daily ritual can be reinforced by performing it at the same time every day—perhaps after your first or second cup of tea or coffee. Include actions that power you up, inspire you, and that anchor you into a positive expectation mindset. With practice and curiosity, you'll find what works for you!

Money Mindset and Prosperity Consciousness

Once you have established a solid set of self-care practices, the next step in cultivating Inner Game is to develop your Money Mindset and Prosperity Consciousness. Have you ever noticed how the taboos around money and sex are eerily similar? Just as people can be held back from authentic sexual expression by shame and social scripts, sexuality professionals and sex coaches often carry beliefs and scripts about money that get in the way of building a thriving private practice. Prosperity Consciousness is developed through a set of specific practices that form your pathway to freedom from these limiting beliefs.

Prosperity Consciousness is how you really look at money, wealth, and abundance in your life, whether personally or through the lens of your business. Prosperity Consciousness encompasses your belief system about money, wealth, and rich people and how these beliefs affect you and keep showing up as your experience increases. The way you think about and relate to money will dictate how you and money get along and how much money you bring in, keep, and put into circulation. If you think money is evil or dirty, guess what? You're going to avoid it. If you think there is a limit to how much money there is, you will be limited.

Four Questions to Reflect on Your Prosperity Consciousness

1. What does money mean to you?
2. What does it mean to you to have money? What does it mean to you to not have money?
3. What's the material purpose or outcome of having money? Buying a house? Having a reliable car? Vacation in Bali?
4. What's the emotional purpose or outcome of having money? To feel more empowered? To achieve financial freedom? To feel joy?

Despite the narratives you project onto money, the simple fact is money itself is neutral. Fundamentally, money is energy that can be put to use toward a variety of ends. Money energy tends to amplify what already is— when applied with the intent to help, money energy multiplies impact, when applied with the intent to harm, money energy amplifies exploitation. To get the most from your money, you need to anchor into the flow of money circulation. Money is constantly in flow and there is power in the cycle of giving and receiving. Keeping your money in circulation is actually part of being prosperous. Practically, this means adopting a mindset of gratitude when getting paid and also when spending money. Focusing on what you're grateful for takes you out of a Lack Mentality.

The Lack Mentality that so many people have doesn't come from a vacuum. Your sense of prosperity or lack is the result of a combination of attitudes, beliefs, values, and life experiences. Together, these attitudes, beliefs, values, and life experiences create your financial thermostat, or your capacity for wealth. Your financial thermostat is a measure of how much money you think you deserve and where you believe money and wealth come from. Put another way, your individual financial thermostat is intimately connected to your sense of worthiness. Consider how much money you made for each of the last three years. Notice if there's a trend. The money you've called in before often serves as a mental benchmark, as well as a symptom of your underlying mindset.

Something to start doing today regardless of where you are with your financial thermostat is to show up for yourself and your business from a position of abundance. Act "as if" regarding money and wealth. Wear objects that connote a philosophy of abundance: pearls, gold, beautiful jewelry, or clothing suited to your body type. Be generous with money. Don't make decisions from lack or need. Practice recognizing all the ways that there is enough to go around. Intentionally notice the abundance all around you—take yourself out of your home or office and experience prosperity in action. Immerse yourself in places like a botanical garden, a posh department store, a grand cathedral bedecked in gold, or any place that is an example of abundance and wealth. If you want to challenge yourself, go to an expensive restaurant and order from the left side of the menu. It can be any meal or an appetizer or just a drink. Do NOT look at the prices on the right or wherever they appear. Order what you want! Indulge yourself. Feel how wealthy you are to not have to worry about how much it costs. Notice how this makes you feel.

Money Attraction

With the basic principles of prosperity consciousness in place, you are ready to begin the next piece of your Inner Game work: Money Attraction. The Inner Game work of Money Attraction builds on your Prosperity Consciousness to enhance your capacity for wealth and keep you energetically connected to the flow of money. It's so important that, if right now what you see in your business and bank account is not enough, you don't get stuck in what is before you. It's where you were before that created where you are right now. You're going to move, just like in sex coaching or the dynamic therapy process, from the present to the future. What you send out into the Universe now is what you will call into your life and business going forward.

Instead of getting stuck in what is, focus on what you want! When you focus on what you want, your mind will shift its attention to solving for your desires. In an oversimplified way, this is the basic neurological underpinning of the Law Of Attraction and the Law Of Allowing. Make the decision to get out of your own way and become open to the limitless possibilities for money to flow to you. Many people look for a direct response when it comes to giving and receiving money: the idea that input A results in output B. However, reality is often much less linear. Remember that you are always making deposits into the bank of the Universe and the returns will come back to you from several different sources.

Britton's MEBES© model, used for holistically understanding a client's sexuality, is also an excellent model for exploring the total life impact you want your money to have. MEBES© stands for Mind, Emotions, Body (and Body Image and Body Behaviors), Energy, and Spirit. Get specific about what you want your money to do for you. The more specific you can be, and the more clearly you can put that intention out into the Universe, the easier it will be to attract the money you want into your life. Use the MEBES© model as a guide to get curious about what's truly at the core of your wanting money, wealth, and prosperity. Dig deep and discover your why.

MEBES© Questions for Money Attraction

Mind: What mental and intellectual needs in your life and business will this money meet?

Emotion: What emotional needs in your life and business will this money meet? What do you want to feel when you have this money?

Body: What physical, bodily needs in your life and business will this money meet?

Energy: What energetic needs in your life and business will this money meet? Where will this money impact your flow?

Spirit: What spiritual needs in your life and business will this money meet?

Financial Stewardship

The final element of your Inner Game work is developing a sound sense of financial stewardship and financial awareness in your life and business. Financial stewardship may involve things like bank statements, spreadsheets, and numbers and is intimately connected to how you think about and relate to money. Your belief system about money influences and directs the decisions you make about financial management. Your prosperity consciousness and money mindset manifest in reality through your financial stewardship. Building greater financial awareness allows you to make better decisions.

Ultimately, financial stewardship is an exercise in prioritization. Your values are the best guide and support for you in this ongoing process of deciding where to invest or spend lavishly, and where to cut back or minimize. The more clearly you can articulate your values, the better a guide they will be. What matters the most to you in your life at large? Authenticity? Family? Autonomy? Honesty? Social justice? Take a look at a list of values and notice which resonate with you at a deep level. For the most potent effect, choose three to five values to prioritize. When you organize your finances to be clearly in integrity with your highest and most cherished values, you'll experience a greater ease and purpose in your working life. When you know your money will allow you to experience the things you care about most, you will remain motivated on the journey ahead.

You interact with money every day. The day-to-day use of money in your life is the perfect learning lab to practice the skills of financial awareness and management. Your daily use of money is real, current data, and your daily needs, wants, and desires need to be met by your business. Also, as a solo-preneur, you are the business. This means many of the expenses that go into maintaining you will be business expenses in the near future if not already. You must structure your business to cover your life.

Financial stewardship requires you to have an awareness of your current financial position and a plan of action going forward. You need to know which accounts you have, your actual outgoing expenses each month, your regular income streams each month, any periodic streams of income you receive, and any debts you may have, including credit cards, loans, or mortgages. Next, create a financial action plan to keep you accountable and get to where you want to be. You want your financial action plan to serve your highest good and bring your financial life in alignment with your values and desires. Your financial action plan needs to account for spending, security, and long-term goals.

Planning for spending, security, and long-term goals is an indispensable part of self-care as an entrepreneur. As an entrepreneur, there are a number of expenses you may have not been responsible for before. For example, you need to plan for self-employment taxes, other taxes, retirement savings, liability insurance, sick leave, and vacation, all of which may have previously been managed by your employer. You need to plan for uneven cash flow by establishing a reserve of savings. You will have decisions to make about whether or not to take on debt as you develop your business, where it is important to understand how debt will impact your ability to make decisions going forward. Finally, you need your efforts to connect back to the Big Whys you have discovered through your Inner Game work in the form of savings toward the experiences and things you yearn to bring into your life. In addition to Inner Game work, the next section focuses on Outer Game and the need for effective implementation.

Outer Game and Effective Implementation

Business is more than passion. At some point, if you want to be successful, you need to turn your business dreams into reality. In the Business of Sex Coaching, this is done by building and strengthening Outer Game: action-oriented approaches that help you step proudly into your role as a smart, efficient entrepreneur. Outer Game is where you work with implementation and manifestation in your business, where you break out of *analysis paralysis* and get things done. The dynamic process of bringing your practice into being starts here with strategic planning for success.

Strategic Planning for Success

Effective Outer Game begins with strategic planning for success: a focus on the nuts and bolts of planning, designing, and creating the template for a successful business. Strategy is like a lighthouse, a beacon to help you keep navigating to where you want to go. Building a private practice is often a bit like being at sea. It's generally not a linear process. There will be storms and you might spot an island that looks really interesting that you want to head off course to explore. As you move through the practice building journey, you can always look to your strategy to reorient you.

Strategy is long-term, high-level, and differentiating. At a minimum, you want to create a strategy focusing on a timeframe of one year, though it's also helpful to encapsulate a bigger vision and take a five-year or ten-year view. Working with your strategy is a chance to look at the high-level picture. It's common for new sexuality professionals to get bogged down in the immediate, urgent details of the day-to-day grind. There is so much to do, and you're likely to be doing all or most of it yourself. Strategic planning is a chance to step back from the fray and gain perspective. The best strategy leans into what makes you different. There are a number of ways you can differentiate yourself, including your unique take on the work (sex coaching or other modalities), your unique approach in your private practice, or the specific audience or sexual concern that you are best placed to serve.

Fundamentally, strategy is all about the choices you make as you build your business. As an entrepreneur, you've got limited resources. Your day has 24 hours and you live in a human body that needs rest, leisure, sleep, and connection in addition to your working time. You have a limit to how much money, energy, sleep, and time you can invest before you need to replenish. Rather than trying to do it all (and burning out in the process), the role of your strategy is to contain your business within a set of tempering constraints—boundaries and limitations that make the whole stronger. With your strategy prepared, you will be ready to face, without becoming overwhelmed, the avalanche of decisions that just keep coming in the life of a business owner.

There are many approaches to strategic planning. The Business of Sex Coaching uses a template for a business strategy plan that brings your mission, vision, purpose, and core values together with a SWOT (strengths, weaknesses, opportunities, threats) analysis, strategic goals, objectives, actions, and benchmarks. Your mission is what drives you, and it's the broadest way to describe what you uniquely do and for whom. Your vision is what you aspire to in a big picture, how-the-world-will-be-different way. Your purpose is what guides you and it's why you're in business in practical terms. Your core values keep you accountable and explain how you do business.

Your SWOT analysis grounds you in the strengths, weaknesses, opportunities, and threats related to both you and your business. Your strategic goals focus your energy and outline how you will use your mission to achieve your vision. Your objectives and actions are what move your dreams into reality. Your objectives are what you will do by when and your actions are how you will implement them. Finally, your benchmarks are your early warning system that help to keep you on course. As you remain on course, you will find that your expertise or niche begins to become more salient in the work that you do as well as attract your ideal clients and customers.

Your Niche: Ideal Clients and Customers

A strategic priority for every sexuality professional building a private practice is to be crystal clear about the clients you are best placed to serve. After creating a big picture business strategy plan, the Business of Sex Coaching focuses next on developing an in-depth understanding about your ideal clients and customers. Your knowledge of your niche will be one of your main points of differentiation and therefore will inform everything you do when marketing your services. Just as your clients are at the heart of your sessions, so they should also be at the heart of your business. When you're not sure what products or services to offer, returning to your potential clients and their wants, needs, hopes, and fears will help you to choose wisely.

The process of identifying and getting to know your ideal clients can be challenging. After all, the work that goes into understanding your ideal clients and customers is the foundation of your marketing efforts. The good news is you have more skills than you realize that are transferable to this process. Getting to know your ideal clients is less about using the perfect formula or following an exact process and is much more about empathy, kindness, compassion, and understanding. The best marketing is a form of emotional labor that requires you to listen deeply to the pains, fears, hopes, and dreams of those you wish to serve. One of your duties as a healer is to make it possible for those that need your help to find you. Knowing who your people are is part of how you do exactly that.

First, narrow down who it is that you would like to serve in your practice. As a clinician, you're trained to address many types of sexual concerns across the life cycle for people from a wide range of gender identities, sexual orientations, and lifestyle choices. But, as the saying goes, "If you try to appeal to everyone, you appeal to no one." By identifying your niche in detail, you'll be able to communicate with your ideal clients and customers in their own words, which helps them quickly identify that you understand them and their concerns.

You need to consider your passion, your interests, and the people who show up for you when defining your niche. Your passion matters because your commitment to the change you want to create in the world will see you through the inevitable challenges you will face along the way. Having a strong interest in the sexual concerns and types of people you will be working with is essential to maintain the effort and attention it takes to build a thriving practice. Factoring in who naturally shows up for you is important because it is far easier to build a blockbuster practice when there is demand from your audience. Once you've considered your passion, interests, and who shows up, take a look at the intersection of these three elements. Where all three overlap, that's where you'll find your niche!

Questions to Help Define Your Niche

Your Passion

1. What is your "calling" or what are you really good at?
2. What are you passionate about?
3. What fires you up or gets you really excited?
4. What do you wish would change in the world, in society, or in people's lives?

Your Interests

1. Which sexual concerns or client types captivate you and hold your interest?
2. Which topics related to sexuality can you just not seem to find enough materials to study further?
3. What types of talks or workshops do you not hesitate to attend?
4. What sessions do you choose to go to if you're at a conference about sexuality?

Who Shows Up for You

1. What kind of people have you noticed coming to you to ask you about sexuality?
2. Who comments on your social media posts?
3. Who comes up to you at networking events or parties to ask you more?
4. Who reaches out to you and what do people typically ask you to share?

Your niche and your ideal client type will change over time, so don't stress about finding the perfect niche. After all, there's no such thing as perfect! As a case in point, even Britton's ideal client has shifted over time! When she established her private practice in 1993, she was collaborating with Betty Dodson and primarily serving preorgasmic women. She also had a column in a weekly New York newspaper that attracted a lot of different client types. She began to shift away from just serving preorgasmic women to serving whoever showed up. In the process, she became a specialized generalist in sexology. But when she began developing her personal website, drpattibritton.com, Britton knew she needed to get more specific. That project helped her identify four niches, which narrowed over time to just three: older virgin males, especially in tandem with a surrogate partner therapist, older people working with sexuality and aging, and sexless couples.

Once you've got your niche, the next step is to create a client avatar that represents your ideal client in a great degree of detail. A client avatar has four parts: a client profile, their felt needs, their decision-making process, and alternatives, a.k.a. the competition. A client profile captures demographic information about your ideal client as well as where they go for information when they're looking for answers. Your ideal client's felt needs relate to their deep sense of identity and how that will impact what they need in order to choose to work with you. Your ideal client's decision-making process includes the steps they follow to decide to work with you, including their financial process and whether or not they need approval from a partner. Finally, you need to know the alternatives to working with you that your ideal client is considering

It's not enough to know who your ideal clients are. You also need to speak their language: to describe their challenges and desires back to them in their own words. When your ideal clients hear themselves in your marketing, they will feel heard and understood, which, in turn, cultivates trust. You can get a preliminary feel for the language your ideal clients use by reading their words online, for example in book reviews, forums, and the comment section of the videos they are watching. Then, the best way to capture the language your ideal client uses is to spend some time talking to them directly! Conduct a series of interviews with people from your niche to explore the challenges they face, the outcomes they're looking for, and how you uniquely may be able to help them. In both instances, you want to capture how your ideal clients speak about themselves and their challenges, word-for-word, in their own words. These words will become the targeted marketing copy for selling your programs, services, or products. The products that you develop (productizing) and your capacity to generate revenue and profits from those products (monetizing) may serve as a launching opportunity for your business.

Productizing and Monetizing

In-depth knowledge of who you will serve in your practice will also allow you to take your skills and competency as a sex coach, as well as your unique gifts, and turn these into products and service offerings that pay. The next step in your Outer Game work is to create what are termed as "offers" such as programs, products, and one-to-one services: these are the elements of your business that are of great value to your ideal clients and customers, ones that monetize your message and that are priced so you can thrive. For many Business of Sex Coaching students, productizing and monetizing can feel very exciting but also scary and overwhelming at times. Don't be surprised if your "stuff" comes up in the process—creating and pricing offers is one place where Inner Game and Outer Game heavily overlap. When that happens, remember to pace yourself, step it out, and keep your eye on the prize of a thriving sex coaching business as you go through this process.

We no longer live or work in a time where you are only a coach or a therapist, where you're just there to help your clients reach their stated goals. To build a practice that endures, you need to productize and monetize your work, which includes branding, marketing, and sales. Productize means to create marketable products with the aim of producing income. Products aren't just things, products can be physical objects, services, or a combination of both. Monetize means to convert your message into something saleable and to set a price for what you offer. Today's global marketplace is full of sophisticated consumers with high expectations who have the ability to choose from a huge range of possible solutions to their problems. While that can seem intimidating at first, there's also a thrill and a joy and an aliveness to the marketplace that you will tap into as you become a part of it. Productizing your client work and going beyond the talk session is exciting, creative, and gives you leverage to add more.

Your products are ultimately what produce revenue, that is, products yield income. Your suite of products can include one-to-one or group bundles, packages or programs, sex toys and other pleasure products, lectures, seminars, classes, workshops, retreats, affiliate products, endorsements, and even sliding fee scale sessions, among others. This list isn't exhaustive, but rather just to whet your appetite and get your creative juices flowing! When it comes to bundles, packages, and programs, generally bundles are multiples of the same product, often at a discount compared to the one-off price, whereas packages or programs are generally made up of several different products put together. To use a fruit analogy, bundles are like bags of peaches and packages are like several different fruits together in your fruit basket.

Pricing

You can have all the products in the world, but if you can't sell them, you're not running a business… you've got a hobby. Monetization is what makes your business REAL. When you monetize your message, you hone the message that gets you up in the morning and that deeply resonates with your ideal clients, and then translate that through to product pricing, whatever the product may be. There are nearly endless ways you can approach setting prices. The method used in the Business of Sex Coaching is to work out a unique pricing baseline to Ensure you meet all of your needs and then some to allow for growth. Your unique pricing baseline is the minimum amount you need to generate from every live paid hour of work you do. It can also be helpful to be familiar with the pricing of other similar practitioners who are local to the clients that you serve. While you want to move away from selling coaching or therapy hours like commodities, having this in mind serves as a starting point grounded in math rather than emotion.

It takes time and intentional effort to get a butt in a seat whether it's a workshop, a training, a webinar, or a one-to-one client. For every one paid hour (be that in a client session, delivering a retreat, or running a workshop), there's anywhere from two to ten hours of marketing, administration, preparation, and follow-up. A powerful way to maximize the returns you receive from the unpaid hours of energy and labor you pour into your business is through packages, bundles, and programs. You can bring together a suite of products or a bundle of sessions to fully address one of your ideal client's points of pain. This way, you can work together with someone over a longer period of time rather than on a one-off, à la carte basis, which helps with cash flow and securing commitment to the work.

There's no right way to decide whether to create bundles, packages, or programs. Bundles tend to be made up of multiple sessions, for example, four-session, eight-session, or twelve-session bundles. Generally, bundled sessions are sold at a discount compared to the one-off session price. Packages and programs, on the other hand, often bring together sessions with other products and services. For example, you could offer a three-month program that includes six sessions, access to an online course, email support in between sessions, access to a private podcast feed, and your signature eBook. Each has advantages and disadvantages. For example, packages and programs can be confusing for some clients, whereas bundles are often easier to understand. Packages and programs can sometimes feel overwhelming to set up, especially if you're just starting out, whereas bundles are simpler to create. On the other hand, bundles can result in price shopping or having clients reduce their perception of value down to the hourly rate rather than the results they will experience. Packages and programs are much harder to reduce to an hourly rate, because they include different types of products. Bundles tend to be more general in their application, whereas packages and programs can be tailored to hot button client concerns. Educational product development may be an essential asset for sex coaches to develop thriving practices.

Educational Product Development

The first product most emerging sex coaches and sexuality professionals create and sell is an educational product—a talk, a workshop, a seminar, or a class. In the Business of Sex Coaching, students are challenged to create, market, sell, and deliver an educational product at this point in their Outer Game work. One of the best things about educational products is that, unlike in-depth one-to-one or group work, *you do not need to be a certified professional to deliver them.* For this reason, educational products are excellent early income generators and a solid path to build your confidence as both a sexuality professional and as an entrepreneur.

Educational products are anything where you deliver a message in a structured way to other people. The message can be delivered in person or virtually, live or asynchronously, such as an online course or webinar recording. You can deliver the message unidirectionally, like in a talk or lecture, where you share information and attendees receive it. You can have a two-way exchange of information, like in the case of a workshop, where you share information and elicit response and interaction from participants. Or, depending on whether or not you are qualified to do so, you can train others to carry on and present the message, as is the case when training other professionals.

Designing and Leading a Successful SAR

Sexual Attitude Reassessment & Restructuring (SAR) training is a pivotal sensitivity training in the field of sexology. The world badly needs more people who are competent to create and lead SAR and, what's more, SAR is a powerful professional training educational product to add to your product suite. The first and so far only comprehensive guide to developing your own SAR is *Designing and leading a Successful SAR: A guide for sex therapists, sexuality educators, and sexologists* by Dr. Patti Britton and Dr. Robert Dunlap, published by Routledge.

To create a transformative educational product, you must account for the ways people learn and the different learning domains. There are three primary ways that people learn: through the eyes, the ears, or the body. You want to create educational products that address all three learning styles: you want to show them things, you want them to hear things, and you want them to experience and feel things. There are also three learning domains: cognitive, affective, and experiential. The cognitive is the thinking domain. The affective is the feeling, emotional domain. The experiential is the behavioral domain. Include all three domains—get your students to think, feel, and do—into any product you design and deliver for maximum impact.

Even the simplest of educational products benefits from thoughtful curriculum design. Curriculum design means everything that goes into building a structure for your educational product. To build your curriculum, you must decide which pieces and elements you will include and in what order. That said, the best curriculum design is subtle, it's as much art as it is pedagogical science. When you think about creating your curriculum, think about being a composer writing music or an artist painting a mural, rather than an engineer making precise calculations. Just as artists hone their craft over time, you're going to improve at curriculum design the more you do it. Before you know it, it will come to you naturally as part of your expertise!

You need more than a beautifully designed curriculum to help your students get results. You also need to actively develop group leadership skills. To be a group leader, whether you're giving a talk, leading a workshop, or you're a trainer, you have to possess several important qualities. You have to have polished public speaking skills, including time management skills, to effectively and clearly deliver your message. You need to develop poise under duress because things are going to go wrong. You also have to be ready when emotions appear, like anger, sadness, or other deep emotional states, to welcome those emotions and to honor the process. You have to know how to process a group through facilitation, development, and trouble spotting. You have to be present-centered to feel what's going on in your group and be prepared to make adjustments if something won't work in terms of how you planned it. Finally, you need to be able to hold the attention of your group, which is most easily achieved by being dynamic, energetic, and engaging.

The best way to develop group leadership skills and to improve your abilities as an educator is to practice, practice, practice! You can practice speaking in front of a mirror which, while it might sound a little ridiculous, is some of the best preparation for feeling comfortable seeing your own face while teaching on Zoom. Go to other people's events and practice being an observer where you read into what's going on and notice the dynamics in the room. Take frequent opportunities to practice being a listener. Practice being courageous in every area of your life—the best group leaders can hear, sense, and feel what is going on and are daring enough to name it.

WDYD

Once the basic foundations of your private practice are in place, the next step is to spread the word far and wide about what you do. The Business of Sex Coaching approaches this challenge by guiding students to craft a signature speech, one that answers the pivotal question that drives all of your marketing: "What Do You Do (WDYD)?" As a sex coach or sexuality professional, you need to be able to articulate the seven elements of what you do in a variety of contexts, from a one-minute elevator pitch to an elongated response that could form the basis of an entire workshop or training.

The 7 Elements of the What Do You Do Speech

1. Your Name and Credentials: Name as you want to be known—degrees, certifications, achievements, awards, etc.
   a. Credibility—What makes you an expert at what you offer?
   b. Vulnerability—What have you overcome that lends value to your work?
2. Your Position or Professional Identity: Who are you in the marketplace?
3. Your Target Audience/Your Niche: Who do you serve?
4. The "Points of Pain" that you resolve: What challenges, obstacles, or issues can you help them to resolve?
5. The Benefits/Results: What results do you offer and bring to your target audience?
6. The Features: Talk about your programs or services—How they work.
7. Your Call to Action: Your gift or offer. Be sure to tell them what you want them to do!

The WDYD answer draws from everything covered so far in the Business of Sex Coaching. You need to be clear on the primary benefits of your work that address your ideal client's pressing needs, your credentials and credibility, your program features, your target niche, and the action you want people to take. The truth is that most people aren't polished at conveying what they do in a way that captures the true depth of the value they bring in the most impactful way for the audience they're speaking to. In fact, many people just start talking about whatever comes to mind when asked what they do, which doesn't serve them or the person asking, and certainly not their business. Mastering the WDYD answer is going to pivot you to become successful and attractive to your client and customer base.

Anywhere that anybody asks you, what do you do, you need to have an answer that fits in the time available. Your flexible WDYD answer can be brief or you can use it as a whole day workshop. This is known as the accordion effect. For example, maybe it's an elevator speech… literally in an elevator! Maybe you're at a networking event and you have a certain number of seconds to sell what's going on in your private practice. Maybe you have the opportunity to give a talk at a conference or to give a lecture and you have one to two minutes at the beginning to introduce yourself. Or maybe you have the luxury of an all-day workshop where you can stretch out your WDYD as its own presentation. Being able to expand or contract your WDYD answer accordingly is an important skill in its own right.

Sample "What Do You Do?" Speech

Hello, my name is Dr. Patti Britton, Clinical Sexologist, pioneering sex coach, and the co-founder of Sex Coach U, the premier sex coach training and certification organization in the world. I help therapists, coaches, healers, medical professionals, and others who are struggling to be taken seriously, get the right training, and live their most passionate calling.

What I find is that often they want credibility, competency, a thriving business, and a community of support. Our rigorous Business of Sex Coaching program enriches the journey for aspiring sexological entrepreneurs to find their footing, learn what to know and be able to do, and thrive as professionals.

I'd be happy to offer you a one-time Complimentary 1:1 BOSC Discovery Session. Click on the URL to learn more: https://bit.ly/GetBOSC

Practice builds confidence in presenting yourself and what you do. Presenting yourself when you run the business and you are the business can feel daunting. It's normal to feel wobbly and incompetent about this in the beginning… all of us do! Your sense of confidence will grow through regular, repeated rehearsal. Take every opportunity you can to practice sharing who you are and what you do with warm crowds—with professional colleagues, family, friends, or anyone who can serve as a safe space. You will keep changing what you say as you refine your message and your offers, and as you learn to better read and speak to a given audience. Over time, your What Do You Do answer becomes a response that comes from deep within, polished and rehearsed to the point where it feels normal and natural. Potential clients need to be able to easily locate you and your expertise. Web presence is an essential element needed for your sex coaching business.

Web Presence

Being able to accurately describe what you do and leverage a compelling presence is a key part of the next step in Outer Game: developing your web presence. In the Business of Sex Coaching, understanding the general themes about your presence online can become a large part of your overall business success. Your web presence needs to connote, denote, and send out to the world a compelling energy to call people in to learn more about you and your business. What's important is to look at web presence from all its dimensions and to remember that there is no one-size-fits-all list of what you must do for your web presence. You only need to show up online in a way that works for you to better reach your ideal clients and customers. For some of you, that might even mean that you don't need any web presence at all!

If you take away only one thing when it comes to web presence, let it be to Keep It Simple, Sweetie (KISS). The KISS method will save you frustration, headache, and overwhelm as you go about showing up on the Internet. You can keep it simple by approaching your web presence strategically. First, decide on the purpose of your web presence. For example, you may want your web presence to attract clients, to generate media inquiries, to serve as a calling card for a book deal or a Netflix original series, or to drive participation and signups for your events. Next, think about what you like to do online and your level of comfort with technology and the Internet. For example, if you feel comfortable on Instagram or Facebook, or if you prefer reading long-form copy over at Medium, these are things to notice. Finally, you need to identify where the audience you want to reach online can be found, be they prospective clients, journalists, or publishers. You only need to go where the people you want to reach are. By considering purpose, personal comfort, and your audience, you can narrow your activities and become very selective about the web presence you develop.

Once you've created a strategy, then you can start thinking about tactics and finding the right tools to fulfill your purpose and meet your clients where they are. It's common for new sex coaches and sexuality professionals to feel pressure to show up everywhere—a website, a YouTube channel, a podcast, a Twitter, Facebook pages and groups, an Instagram account, on and on and on. Stop! That way leads only to frustration and overwhelm. Instead, go through your strategy-focused priorities and pick your top three web presence platforms. Yes, only three! You have permission to only focus on your top three and release the idea that you need to do it all or get it all done. Remember, if one platform you've chosen doesn't work, that's fine! You can leave it and pick something else to give a try.

Believe it or not, you're now ready to construct your online world! It's important to remember that when potential clients interact with your content online, you're not there in person. You're not in a room giving a talk where you can address people's questions. People are passing by and you don't even necessarily know they're there. To create and nurture asynchronous relationships, you need to make sure your online content reflects the 3 R's: that it is Relevant, Resonant, and creates Results. You make your content relevant when you answer your ideal client's questions about their concerns through the media they enjoy consuming. You make your content resonant by using the language that your ideal clients use, so that they can see themselves in your writing and walk away feeling deeply understood.

Finally, you demonstrate that you create results by offering a quick, direct solution to a bite-sized problem your ideal client has. Often, but not always, this will be in the form of a lead magnet. A lead magnet is something of value you offer when someone joins your mailing list. Remember, lists are the gold of any online business. Lead magnets can include things like checklists, eBooks, webinars, quizzes, email trainings, or challenges, among others. The possibilities for lead magnets are endless. In this exchange of value, you answer a question, solve one small problem, or address one small challenge in exchange for an email address. When it comes to lead magnets, you can use the KISS method, too. Use the tools you have accessible right now to present something attractive to your audience. For example, instead of worrying about how to create a beautifully formatted PDF with fillable fields, you can create a lead magnet in Google Docs and simply deliver it as a Google Doc. If you keep it simple, you can get it up, running, and out very fast. From there, while your lead magnet is already hard at work attracting your ideal clients, you can iterate behind the scenes.

You also want to sculpt a web presence that builds trust at every opportunity. You can strengthen trust with your potential clients online through consistency, credibility, and timeliness. Consistency means being a predictable presence online and can include reaching your audience by regularly releasing content and using a similar brand voice in your presentation across platforms. Credibility in this context means making it easy to determine that your business is legitimate. You check for the credibility of what you discover online all the time. Say you've discovered a business. You want to do your due diligence and avoid fraud. You might check the business's social media accounts to see if there are any recent posts or check the publication date on the newest blog post. When you can see a business is active and that there's somebody there, it's reassuring. Timeliness is staying up to date, not getting stale, and tracking trends in the industry, for example the rise of video to communicate and connect, or increased accessibility provisions like closed captions.

Speaking of industry trends, there are some unique challenges that come with being a sex coach or sexuality professional online that you need to keep in mind. It can be especially hard, when you are fighting for sexual rights and freedoms, to consider censoring the language that you use in your brand name or URL choice. The thing is, using the word sex or even some concepts around sex, sexuality, and eroticism can be like putting up a red flag that attracts extra scrutiny, makes you a target for attacks on your website, or gets email sent directly to the spam folder. You may also struggle for your posts to be visible on certain social media platforms if your brand name or content violates the terms of service. You have to be careful. Be mindful to avoid sexual slang terms in your URL or brand name. You can always use your own name or a more benign approach for your overarching brand name and URL, then offer a special event or program or package that sizzles with sexually charged language within the front-facing pages of your website.

At the same time, there can be real advantages to using the word sex. Depending on your ideal clients, sex can be very clear in sending the right messaging more than other word choices. Using sex in your brand name or URL also has a degree of search relevance. For example, if someone searches for "sexuality" or "sex coach" but you've replaced sex with the word intimacy, you are less likely to get found through that passing traffic. Having sex in your brand can also be beneficial on some of the more sex positive online platforms like PleazeMe, Medium, and Twitter. In crowded online spaces, sometimes you stand out if you've got a brand that has sex in the name. Ultimately, you have to make a pragmatic decision while still owning what it is that you do.

Although not all sexuality professionals need a website as part of their online presence, there are advantages to owning a little bit of your own online real estate, rather than building on the borrowed land of platforms owned by others. If you decide to create a website, keep it simple by beginning with just four pages: Home, About, Services, and Contact. Identify only one action per page that you would like a visitor to take and keep that as the focus as you build each page. Your Homepage communicates to the world what your website is about and invites folks who visit to join your newsletter. Your About page introduces who you are in a way that is in service to your potential clients and invites readers to visit your Services page. Your Services page is essentially where you lay out what you offer and invite visitors to book a discovery call or otherwise take the first action in working with you. Finally, your Contact page spells out how someone can reach you and invites visitors to get in touch. Keep your contact page easy to read, and free of jargon, and it will serve as a good landing location as you market your practice, expertise, and services. The next section expounds upon marketing implementation and launching your business.

Marketing Implementation and The Launch

With your web presence in place, you're ready to bring everything you have done together and send it out into the world to implement your marketing and launch your practice, products, programs, or services. In the Business of Sex Coaching, it is incredibly important that sexuality professionals learn to market with joy, rather than resistance or fear. A lot of people go, "Oh, marketing! I hate marketing!" and associate marketing with being creepy, pushy, or misleading. While that is how some businesses choose to market, you can make different choices. Simply put, marketing is actually attraction in action. Marketing is the relational alchemy of the actions you take in the messages you send out to attract prospective customers and invite them into your business. As is true elsewhere in BOSC, the KISS method applies to your marketing implementation as a whole to keep it from becoming overwhelming.

Everything that you've done up until now will be brought to bear in your marketing implementation, especially and including your Inner Game work.

When emerging sexuality professionals first address marketing, they often experience fear of rejection, fear of being judged, fear of failure, self-doubt, perfectionism, or Imposter Syndrome. Marketing can bring to the surface the old messages and beliefs you carry, like not being good enough or smart enough. Ultimately, this is because being a great marketer requires you to be vulnerable. Vulnerability is actually where power lies, because when you allow yourself to be vulnerable, you're risking it all and nobody can really take anything away from you.

While it may come as a surprise, you have ample skills that transfer to marketing, because sexuality professionals know a thing or two about what it means to navigate vulnerability in pursuit of authentic self-expression. One powerful way to reframe marketing to an area of competence is to use a *dating metaphor*. There are elements of flirting and teasing with your audience when you're marketing. Marketing involves playful interaction where there's some intent and interest, and also some back and forth. The interaction is warm but with something still hidden and held back. There's mystery as you reveal yourself bit by bit, with the occasional invitation to take the next step in the relationship. Finally, for your interactions to feel good and empowering for you and your prospective clients, you need to ground your marketing in consent.

Just like in dating, it's a push-away if you come across as needy. Instead, when you come across as contained within yourself, self-confident, and powerful, without being overly assertive or aggressive, you become attractive. You can choose to hold the bar high and derive your marketing from a place of deep caring for your target audience and your ideal clients. When you are always operating ethically and from a place of consensual engagement, this radiates out into the world in a way that others pick up on. The vibe your marketing puts out is going to affect and infect in a good or a bad way. From this place, you influence how you are received, perceived, and how others respond to you.

This energy carries over to building your audience, too. In order to market your products, services, workshops, or whatever you're offering, you must have people to market to. This means you need to be building an audience right from the beginning, as well as dedicating energy to audience (or list) building as an ongoing business activity. The sooner you get started on building your audience, the better! You need to know where your ideal clients are or think about where you are going to find them. Then, you need to invite them in! Most sexuality professionals, emerging and seasoned alike, fall short when it comes to extending the invitation. Many helping professionals, healers, healthcare workers, or practitioners of the healing arts in general tend to be givers and feel more comfortable being in service. You must learn to avoid the trap where you are always giving and never asking for anything in return. It's not enough to just be present, you have to ask and invite your prospective clients to engage a bit deeper.

Often, the first invitation you will make is to establish a way you can keep in touch. This could include joining your email newsletter, following you on social media, listening to your podcast or radio show, reading your blog or newspaper column, or by connecting in person at a live event. While all of these methods can work to build an engaged audience, it's worth paying special attention to building an email list. Your email list is an asset to your business because you own it. It's great to connect with people where they already are, be that Facebook, Twitter, YouTube, Reddit, or other social media, but you also don't own those platforms. You don't set the rules. Unfortunately, sexuality professionals often run the risk of falling foul of the social media censors. No matter what rules come and go on social media, your email list is yours.

Once you have invited someone into your world, you need to know how you will nurture that connection. The path you guide someone along as you build and deepen a relationship with them is also known as your *funnel*. Here's some good news: funnels don't have to be complicated or follow a specific formula or rigid definition in order to be wildly successful. In the Business of Sex Coaching, a *funnel* is defined as a customer-focused marketing model that illustrates the theoretical journey a customer takes toward the purchase of your product or your service. It's curating the experience someone has with you, where you give them opportunities to opt in and engage more deeply or opt out, if what you are offering isn't right for them.

Continuing with that dating metaphor, engaging your audience is where you nurture these relationships through to the second date and beyond. You engage your audience in four main ways: educate, entertain, surprise, and delight. Educating your audience is specifically about helping them know more about you, what you do, and how to better understand the problems, points of pain, or challenges they are experiencing. Entertaining your audience is about lighting them up and building anticipation about engaging with your content. Surprising your audience is about capturing attention by doing something unexpected. Delighting your audience is about giving them experiences of pleasure. When you incorporate engage, entertain, surprise, and delight into your approach to engaging your audience, you get to have fun conspiring on behalf of the greater good of your potential clients.

When you nurture and deepen relationships with your prospective clients in intentional, thoughtful ways through your content, you help your audience get ready to work with you. When Britton lived in New York City in the early 1990s, she had four clients when she first opened her private practice. At the time, she worked collaboratively with Dr. Betty Dodson, who would send clients over sometimes, but basically, she was starting out fresh with a shiny new Ph.D. in hand. One day, one of Britton's friends gave her the great idea to go to a local throwaway weekly newspaper and offer to do a weekly column for free. After she began writing this column, people would reach out by phone or email. By the time they reached her, they had already read her authentic voice and knew her identity as that sassy sex coach in New York City. When she would ask, "Would you like to talk about how I work?" they would reply, "Oh, no, no, no! I know you."

In this way, nurturing relationships through your content does a lot of the heavy lifting for you, before a prospective client ever makes it to a discovery session. That's because your marketing is your pre-sales. Before you ever get on a sales call, you have the power to prepare your prospective clients in advance. The more your prospect knows about you before they join the call, generally the shorter that call will be. In addition to having your content work for you by nurturing your prospective clients, you can also actively market your products and services by launching them.

The Launch

One powerful option for marketing your products is to launch them: to make an event out of bringing them to market. The Business of Sex Coaching blends the revolutionary systemic Launch framework created by Jeff Walker together with the specific know-how required in order to successfully launch as a sexuality professional. Walker is the originator of the concept of using a Launch to generate new business. In his book,[6] through free videos, workshops, trainings, and elite Launch Club, he teaches how to use the Product Launch Formula (PLF) to rinse, repeat, and reap the rewards.

By transforming your marketing into events, your products, services, and programs can be offered in a new way to your target audience. Once you develop Launch mode thinking, your entire approach to marketing will shift. Everything you have to offer your customers, students, clients, and the world you serve, will now come from the exciting perspective that you are opening a new event for them.

The simple concept of a Launch is based on a three-phased approach: The Pre-Pre Launch, the Pre-Launch, and the Launch. During your launch, you will offer a product, service, or program you wish to sell to your ideal client or customer in a designated period of time, with specific days for opening and closing your payment options. These three phases include the following elements in order to attract prospective buyers:

- Interest building.
- Seeding the launch toward an offering using a Problem/Solution focus.
- Addressing resistance factors.
- Giving high-value content.
- Acknowledging the buyer's needs (points of pain).
- Making the sale to serve the buyer for their promised Transformation (outcome).

In this process of setting up your events, you begin to show the offer and why the customers need it, looking at your own Big Why as your motivation.

You are paving the way for your customers to achieve the transformation you promise. Simple, but not easy! You can tease interest within your target audience through a series of high-value educational or information products, such as email sequences, podcasts, social media posts, or a series of informational videos. By leaning into the release of a new offer, whether it is a low-cost webinar, a new book, or an ongoing professional training program, as you get ready to make it available to your audience, you have a new approach to doing so. Launching can be rewarding in every sense of the word! Once your business is launched, you will need a systematic way to enroll and onboard new clients.

Enrolling and Onboarding New Clients

At this point, the Business of Sex Coaching has covered all of the necessary steps to get you launched and on your way to serving your client base! Now, it's time to learn how to enroll or sell your prospects for your varied products and services. A great deal of finesse is involved in vetting your potential clients and in converting a prospect into a buyer. You need to develop a masterful intake mindset and hone your ability to anticipate and address potential resistance factors, to move the conversation forward, and to secure sales. You can do all of this in a way that feels good, is energetically aligned, and comes from service.

If you're not savvy about how to sell your offers to your ideal clients, you are going to struggle to make money. Regardless of whether you identify as a healer, a helping professional, an educator, a coach, a clinician, or something else besides, you need to have the art of sales mastery if you want to build a private practice that goes the distance. In the Business of Sex Coaching, we look at the entire ecosystem involved in bringing in a new client and break it down into two parts: enrollment and onboarding. *Enrollment* means bringing somebody into your services, including making the sale, collecting payment, and signing the client agreement. *Onboarding* is the process you follow to get a new client started on their journey and orient them to what is to come.

Most emerging sexuality professionals launch their private practices by initially offering one-to-one services. Recognizing this, the Business of Sex Coaching covers an enrollment process that is well-suited to one-to-one sales calls, sometimes also known as discovery calls or initial consultations. Starting with one-to-one work is a powerful way to build your business simply because it is the quickest way to start. That said, you don't have to do sales calls! There are other ways to sell your packages, programs, and educational products including sales pages, webinars, email, text, or through direct messaging on social media platforms. The same core principles apply to all of these different approaches to having sales conversations.

Sales conversations can be challenging for helping professionals, especially for coaches and others using action-oriented modalities, because they differ from the way that you normally interact with your clients. In sales, you focus on the What, not the How. The What encompasses the client's current situation and the scope of work you do. The How encompasses the detailed approach to the client's specific situation, including things like action steps or home assignments. You don't cover the How on a sales call. A common mistake is to give a prospective client so much information and guidance that your prospect walks away happy and feeling like you resolved their problem… and then you can't get anybody to book with you! By sticking to the What, you can avoid this frustrating outcome.

You need to manage your energy and keep your energy high throughout your sales calls. Your energy has a powerful impact because it drives the connection and keeps the conversation flowing. The Business of Sex Coaching approaches this concept as High Vibration Sales, or selling from service. Many people, including your prospective clients, have the impression that selling is manipulative, creepy, or icky. You can turn that around and reframe your energy around sales by deciding that you will be selling from service, where you're in service to your prospective client and to yourself throughout the process. You show up to a sales call for the highest good of the relationship.

Another component of High Vibration Sales is that your sales process has the function of education. Throughout the sales conversation, you're helping your prospective client understand what is possible for them and then upholding that vision so they can see and anchor into it themselves. You will often speak with folks who have a vague idea that they're not happy with something and think maybe you can help. When you are skilled at sales, you will open up their world to new, exciting possibilities and an understanding of what getting there will require. In this way, you can have a profound impact on everyone who joins your discovery calls, whether they choose to work with you or not.

Finally, High Vibration Sales also reframes sales as enrollment. Instead of taking on anyone and everyone, which can often result from approaching sales with a Lack Mentality, you need to consider if a prospective client is qualified. You need to assess if they have the necessary things they need in order to benefit from working with you and going through this process of growth. You need to discover if they are a fit. You need to know if they really are one of your ideal clients, where your work together will be squarely in your areas of strength and expertise. In this way, your enrollment process is an evaluation from both sides. When you don't enroll people who lack the necessary tools to succeed, you are in service to them, to yourself, and to your profession as a whole.

Put another way, effective enrollment requires you to vet prospective clients. Doing a thorough pre-intake is the best way to avoid energy-draining, bad-fit clients. You have to decide whether you want to have prospective clients tell you what's going on ahead of time. You may even decide that prospective clients need to "apply" to work with you. One advantage to having an application, a form they have to fill out, or another screening device is that, often, unqualified prospects will self-select out. If someone isn't willing to invest a few minutes filling out a form, they are less likely to be willing to invest time and money into working with you! You just want to make sure that your vetting process matches up with your ideal client type. Some client types only trust businesses where they can call by phone, even if only to leave a voicemail, whereas others would expect to fill out a form and hop on a Zoom call. You need to consider the needs of both you and your ideal clients.

Once you have your pre-intake or pre-sales process up and running, you are ready to dive into the sales call, or enrollment call, itself! The Business of Sex Coaching uses the OPTIMIZER model to teach how to artfully lead a sales call. The OPTIMIZER model includes the following nine steps: **O**rganize Your Mindset, **P**repare Your Space, **T**imer On for the Call, **I**nitiate, **M**ake Suggestions, **I**ntuit, **Z**one In, **E**mpathize, and **R**einforce the Need for Action. The OPTIMIZER model brings together elements of Inner and Outer Game to form a holistic approach to sales. By getting your mindset and energy right, employing the use of strategic questions, remembering to stick to the What, not the How, and listening deeply, you will sell clients into your offerings with ease and the highest integrity. Be generous, be grateful, and always thank prospective clients for their time. Even if they don't become your client, you're in service to the Universe and humankind.

For those who do enroll into working with you, having a streamlined and comprehensive onboarding process will set your clients up for success. You always want to be guiding your client to the next step. You need to be crystal clear about what happens next because your client is not going to know because they're right at the start of their journey. In order to make sure you've covered everything and to save yourself a lot of time, you can systematize your onboarding process. Create a welcome pack that draws the map for your client and helps them feel calm after making their purchase decision and continues to build trust in your relationship. Just as with any purchase, a client may suffer from Buyers' Remorse. By nurturing them up-front and guiding them with a heavy hand, ala Welcome Pack, they'll feel taken care of as you maximize the likelihood that they feel they are in the right place with you.

Your welcome pack should include everything they need to know and do to take the next steps. Include information about essential logistics, like how to book sessions, where you are meeting, and how communication works outside of sessions. If you haven't already, collect the basic client data you need to serve them, which could include their email address, phone number, or mailing address. You can share the code of professional ethics you follow and information about any professional organizations you are part of to show your professional standards. You also want to include a client agreement and make sure it is signed before you start the first session. You can also gather their sex/relationship history and other intake paperwork you need in advance of your first session. Finally, include any other unique handouts that relate to how you work with clients. Ultimately, systematizing your onboarding process will allow you to scale your practice while

188 *Patti Britton and Sarah Martin*

maintaining a consistent, high-quality experience for all of your clients. The next section addresses some of the strategies and benefits of scaling your practice.

Scaling Your Practice

At this point in the Business of Sex Coaching, everything needed to build a successful practice has been covered. What is the next step beyond success? Growth. As your business grows, you will face new challenges. You can get ready for them now. There is an art and a science to scaling your practice. To continue to grow and expand, you must work on your business, not just in your business. Now more than ever, it is important to consistently and regularly check in with yourself about what you want from your business as you chart the course forward. While you need to consider the next year, the next five years, and the next ten years as you plan to scale, you also want to think about the eventual end game for your business. You may want to pass on your business to your descendants, move into passive ownership, keep it going yourself as long as possible, or sell to new ownership. The approach you take to scaling will vary depending on what you ultimately want.

In order for your business to grow, you need to spend the majority of your time working in your Zone of Genius, a concept first put forward by Hendricks in *The Big Leap* (2010). At any given moment, you are operating in one of four zones: incompetence, competence, excellence, and genius. In your zone of incompetence, many people can do those tasks better than you. In your zone of competence, you're okay at accomplishing those tasks, though you're not doing your best. In your zone of excellence, few people can do those tasks as well as you. The zone of excellence is tricky because it's your comfort zone. It's where people love to pay you for doing these tasks and things seem to come easy. While that may sound nice, in your zone of genius, you are the best in the world. It is from within your zone of genius that you will change the world.

If you're going to scale, most of the time that means your business is going to grow beyond just you. Growing your team can include hiring service providers, independent contractors, or employees, which each have their own set of pros and cons. Regardless of the type of help you bring on board, when you begin to expand your team be sure that your core values drive your hiring. You will also begin developing new skills related to people management and delegation, as well as your own management style. You need to define what it means for you to become the CEO of your business.

You also need to be prepared for the growing pains that come along with developing yourself and really starting to shine as a sexuality professional. The changes that take place during this process won't occur only in your working life—they will ripple out and affect all areas of your life. Your circle of friends will change. The experiences you seek out, the challenges you face, and the problems you have will change. The systems you use in your business, from marketing, to administration, and fulfillment will change, too. This cycle of change never really stops as long as growth continues. As the saying goes, "new level, new devil."

The conclusion of the Business of Sex Coaching program marks the beginning of the next chapter in a student's business life. The way forward is a wide-open road that can lead to wherever you want to take it using all of the knowledge and skills developed throughout this comprehensive curriculum. As you move forward, pause and consider how you will know when you get "there," wherever "there" happens to be for you. Define it, claim it, know it. At the same time, remember that you're never done. Enjoy the journey for what it is. As you move through the challenges and savor the successes, remember that the brighter you can shine your light, the more sexual healing there will be in this world that so desperately needs it. The more successful each of us is, the greater the impact we'll have on the world, to make it a healed, better place.

Conclusions

Too many sexuality professionals fail to build sustainable private practices and other forms of their business to serve their niche or achieve their end-goal career dreams. In order for sexuality professionals to transform the world through greater access to sexual health, sexual rights, and sexual freedoms, it is essential that their time and energy is dedicated to the work of sexology. It is only possible for sexuality professionals to focus on their work if they are sustained and nourished by it. Building successful private practices is absolutely required to bring about widespread sexual healing in our world.

As M. Scott Peck's book, *The Road Less Traveled*, begins, "Life is difficult." Although it is critical for you to employ positive thinking, and to follow powerful role models for moving through the roadblocks that come up in life and business, it isn't always easy. Being an entrepreneur is difficult. It requires knowledge, skills, courage, drive, support, and sustainable energy. In fact, if you revisit the Britton's MEBES© Signature System as your framework for looking at what you need as a successful entrepreneur, it goes like this:

M: Adopt a positive mental mindset about money, prosperity, self-care, attracting the right clients and serving them well, being a smart steward of your business, and being of service to the world.

E: Be the container to which your clients come for healing, clearing, empowerment, knowledge, expertise, practical education, clinically-proven processes, and hope. You need to be the clean, clear emotional container to serve your clients and yourself. Remembering that *you run the business and you ARE the business* is a foundational premise that will help you prioritize and stabilize your decision making for emotional wellbeing.

B: Your body is your own container. You must be a great caretaker and caregiver for keeping your body healthy and well, in all aspects of being human. As a sexological entrepreneur and clinical sexologist, you want to remain in your integrity to *walk your talk*. That means you have healthy erotic and sexual pathways for your personal life that enable you to grow, heal, find joy, experience pleasure, and be fulfilled. The same goes for your business. A business, like a body, needs TLC and the fuel from which to thrive. It also needs to be fun and give you joy!

E: Energy is everything. It is vital to maintain balance, to have sustainable energy reserves, and to find methods in your practice to generate and keep energy alive in your business and in your personal life.

S: Spirit is perhaps the most elusive part of being a sexuality professional who is working as an entrepreneur. What does spirit mean in this context? To know your Big Why—to follow your passion, to honor your commitment to give and receive, to make positive changes in the world, to be of service to others and yourself, and to promote sexual wellness within (and beyond) your own spheres of influence.

There are many inspiring and uplifting possibilities for sexological entrepreneurship, which create an inherent potential for your success. Creating daily habits of success and calling in a community of authentic support will get you through to the Finish Line. What you define as the Finish Line is up to you. Hopefully, you can take away valuable, practical ideas from reading about how sexological entrepreneurs are trained in the Business of Sex Coaching program. You, too, can be a successful sexological entrepreneur.

Questions for Reflection

1. What is one step you can take immediately to improve your business success?
2. What is your single greatest challenge in moving forward toward expanded business success?
3. What is the greatest insight you have gained in reading this chapter that will enrich your potential as a sexuality professional working as an entrepreneur?
4. What do you need to sustain momentum in growing your business knowledge, practical skills, and to empower yourself toward success?
5. What would be the one ingredient that could make or break your ability to succeed as a sexuality professional working as an entrepreneur?
6. From whom would you seek business support? What traits or qualities make them a good entrepreneur to consult?

Notes

1 https://www.aasect.org/continuing-education
2 https://www.sexscience.org/
3 https://worldsexualhealth.net/
4 https://sexcoachu.com/business-of-sex-coaching/
5 See Williams, P., & Davis, D. C. (2007). *Therapist as life coach: An introduction for counselors and other helping professionals.* Norton Professional Books.
6 Walker, J. (2021). *Launch (updated & expanded edition): How to sell almost anything online, build a business you love, and live the life of your dreams.* Hay House Business.

Recommended Resources

Britton, P. O. (2005). *The art of sex coaching: Expanding your practice.* New York: Norton.

Britton, P. O., & Dunlap, R. E. (2017). *Designing and leading a successful SAR: A guide for sex therapists, sexuality educators, and sexologists.* New York, NY: Routledge.

Bundles, A. P. (2020). *Self made: Inspired by the life of madam C.J. Walker.* New York: Scribner, an imprint of Simon & Schuster.

Burchard, B. (2011). *The millionaire messenger: Make a difference and a fortune sharing your advice.* New York: Morgan James Pub.

Eker, T. H. (2019). *Secrets of the millionaire mind: Mastering the inner game of wealth.* Toronto, Ontario, Canada: Collins, an imprint of HarperCollins.

Hancock, J. L. (Director). (2016). *The founder* [Motion picture]. USA: Filmation.

Hendricks, G. (2010). *The big leap: Conquer your hidden fear and take life to the next level.* New York: HarperOne.

McWilliams, P. (1995). *You can't afford the luxury of a negative thought: A book for people with any life-threatening illness–including life (Revised Edition).* Mary Book.

Peck, M. S. (1985). *The road less traveled.* New York, NY: Simon and Schuster.

Rodgers, R. (2021). *We should all be millionaires: A woman's guide to earning more, building wealth, and gaining economic power.* New York, NY: HarperCollins Leadership, an imprint of HarperCollins.

Russell, D. O. (Director). (2015). *Joy* [Motion picture on DVD]. USA: Fox 2000 Pictures.

Walker, J. (2021). *Launch (updated & expanded edition): How to sell almost anything online, build a business you love, and live the life of your dreams.* Hay House Business.

Williams, P., & Davis, D. C. (2007). *Therapist as life coach: An introduction for counselors and other helping professionals.* Norton Professional Books.

13 Beyond Therapy

Entrepreneurship in Sex Therapy Practice

Candice Cooper-Lovett

Introduction

During my doctoral studies, when I completed my dissertation defense and I was announced Dr. Cooper, the first question that was asked was "So what's next?" I had no idea how my journey would unfold upon completing my Ph.D. I had goals of becoming a business owner but I felt it was a far-fetched goal that I would not obtain until I reached my mid-to-late 40s. I became fully licensed at the end of 2013 and six months later, I made the decision to move to Atlanta to further pursue my career. My first job in Atlanta was at a community-based agency where I was clinical director. I realized that this was not something that I was passionate about nor saw doing long term, it was unfulfilling.

Within the first couple of months of moving to Atlanta I met a marriage and family therapist (MFT) at a CEU training who had the same credentials as I. She expressed to me that she was in private practice full-time, and she did not understand why I was not doing the same if that was my goal. I told her I assumed there were a lot of steps involved in starting a private practice and business. In my graduate programs, there was no training on how to become an entrepreneur. The courses primarily focused on becoming a great therapist, a professional, and an academician, but unfortunately there were not many lessons on becoming a business owner. I knew in graduate school that becoming a professor and researcher was not for me.

During my journey into entrepreneurship as a first-generation business owner, there were a lot of lessons I learned over the years. The valuable lesson that I recognized early in my entrepreneurial journey was that I could be the best therapist, and provide the best quality work, however if I didn't know the business of business my company would not flourish. Understanding this has helped me a lot as a therapist and business owner. Since I've started my businesses, colleagues, and past professors have sought me out for consultation and keynote talks focused on starting a private practice. This chapter will discuss the process of starting businesses along with how I incorporated spirituality in my practice.

DOI: 10.4324/9781003314660-13

Creating a Business Plan and Business Location

During the grassroots phase of my business, I was very determined and had the support of great colleagues who were already in business. I also did a lot of research on how to start a successful private practice. During this period, I was working full-time as clinical director and I was intentional about dedicating at least one hour per day after work to develop my business plan. I used Casey Truffo's (2012) be a wealthy therapist book to guide me in creating my business plan. This business plan highlighted the type of practice wanted (solo vs group), where clients are seen, fee structure, sliding scale structure, ideal client, and ideal weekly schedule with clients in the practice. This book served as the foundation of my practice. In the early stages of building my business, I wrote out potential business names, a mission statement, services to be provided, the plans of my business, and distinguishable characteristics that stood out in my practice. Having a guideline of how to develop the practice was a crucial part of my business building process.

Another integral part of my business plan was gaining clarity on the expenses as it related to starting a private practice. I did this by creating a budget system of the baseline necessities that I needed in order to survive (e.g., housing, car expenses, food expenses, and utilities). I deducted what was being spent from the baseline income of my full-time job. I was aware that starting the business in the beginning would incur loss vs gain because it was new.

Additionally, from this budgeting sheet, I had the opportunity to decipher what would be the best pricing for office rent. Based on my budget, I did not want to spend over $500/month. I researched different areas where there was the most need, I recognized the need was on the southside of Atlanta. I found a listing on craigslist where there was an office space for less than my budget of $500/month. As it related to pricing for clients, I did research of therapists in my area with similar credentials, and created pricing that felt affordable for those who would pay out of pocket. Starting off, I charged clients $85 for individual sessions and $125 for couples/family therapy. I also utilized a sliding scale for clients who were unable to afford my therapy rates.

Once those tasks were completed, I began my LLC and completed the Georgia steps to starting a business. In March of 2015, I officially opened the doors to my new practice A New Creation Psychotherapy Services (ANC), where I provided individual, couple and family therapy. ANC has a major focus on transformative growth and stands on the premise that once healing takes place, individuals, couples and families would become a new creation. In 2016, I connected with a sex therapy supervisor, and I began my certification for sex therapy and added that as a service to the ANC practice.

Building the Practice

Since the steps of obtaining an office space and starting the business was completed, the next step was credentialing with insurance panels. I made the choice to have a hybrid practice of self-pay and insurance. I believed that this was a wise choice because I learned from colleagues that insurance companies could assist in providing referrals. In addition, I sent emails to different organizations, hospitals, doctors offices, and crisis centers, that served the clients I wanted to work with. Furthermore, I provided in-services for organizations that allowed me to speak about my practice and what I provided. Additionally, I provided a one paged document of my services, insurances that I accepted, and the type of clients I worked with. Furthermore, I joined various therapist directories to contribute to my business gaining more visibility. I also began a website and started a google business page that was less than $20/month (for the website). I provided information about my services, pricing, the type of clients I work with, and blogs.

When navigating managed care systems and the credentialing process, there were moments of frustration due to paperwork, and lengthy contracts. There were steps of this process that I hadn't learned about. I give credit to the assistance and support of my colleagues to have the ability to navigate managed care systems as a practitioner. In retrospect, it would have been wise to hire someone to do the credentialing process as it can be taxing. Once this step was completed, I was now awaiting the first phone call to book for services. Two months after the start of my business I got my first phone call for a session. From that time, more calls began to come through. At this point, I knew that I needed a part-time assistant to help me with social media marketing and creating a system to engage and interact with clients. I paid my assistant for four hours a week at ten dollars per hour. It made a difference with delegating tasks and getting assistance in creating systems that were useful to the practice. My assistant was also helpful in providing me with resources as it related to branding, head shots, and logos. I got a new logo, and business cards to reflect the tenants of my practice.

Within a year after starting my business, all of my therapy slots were full. I worked 18 client hours per week in addition to my role as clinical director. Years ago, at a business conference I learned that when your business is bringing in the same amount of revenue as your baseline employment, it was time to take the leap. After a year and a half of starting my business and working part-time, I went into full-time private practice in January 2017. Making this decision was one of the scariest and most exciting moments of my life. I was terrified and at times unsure if taking the risk of being a full-time self-employed individual was the right path for me. I participated in a 30-day challenge to take the leap (which meant different things for everyone) and counted down the days to my resignation. During this time, I also saved a lot to have security in case I had slow months in the practice. Upon taking "the leap" I felt a sense of freedom and happiness. I also had some anxiety because I no longer had a consistent check coming in.

I worked in my private practice providing therapy and supervision, and in addition began to do assessments for extra income for community based mental health agencies to offset the weeks where I had a lot of cancellations.

Furthermore, I worked at a university part-time providing supervision to the marriage and family therapy students. At this point in my entrepreneurial journey, I was in a good space with having enough income to sustain my basic living expenses and beyond that. From there, I began to investigate ways of expanding my business.

Adding to the Practice and Branding

When I began to think about expanding my practice, my business coach, who was also my photographer, helped me start my brand and assisted me in organizing my business. The advice given was that I was to not be the face of my business (ANC). I was to allow it to stand on its own, especially with the future goal of having a group practice. ANC would be specific to clients and therapy services. ANC was growing at a pace where I started to provide events for individuals and couples, however I needed my other skill sets such as speaking, supervision, and consultation to be a separate entity from my ANC business. From this point Dr. Coop-Love was created.

In 2019, I launched my consultation business Dr. Coop-Love. I started a website, social media pages, Google business page, and got a Google voice number separate from ANC. This was very helpful in separating my work with speaking, consultation, and supervision from therapy clients. When it came to branding and headshots I updated them every two years to keep my photos relevant and up to date. My business coach would teach me the importance of branding and my style. He shared with me that my style was like a close friend who made people feel comfortable but had professional knowledge to assist them in ways that a friend couldn't.

As it relates to speaking, I have been a mental health speaker for almost 20 years. Often, I'm sought out to be a speaker for different organizations and community networks. I found that speaking was a very lucrative platform, however I struggled with what to charge. My business coach shared with me that I should charge at least $5,000 per talk, however with my personal struggles being humble to a fault, I could not ask for such a price. Although I had been speaking for over 15 years at this point, I did research and asked different colleagues about their price points. I also joined speaker groups to assist me with pricing that was reasonable and felt right for me as a speaker. As for the other branches of the Dr. CL business, I felt it was important to add packages with multiple sessions in a bundle as well as ANC. These services were accessible and could be booked online. These services were to be paid upfront; this avoided a lot of future pitfalls as it related to no-shows and receiving guaranteed pay.

Initially, in addition to speaking, I added supervision services for pre-licensed professionals and consultation services for those interested in starting a private practice. I also added clinical consultation for therapists who were fully licensed and may have difficulties on a clinical case that related to my expertise. At the time, I began to research pricing that was competitive and marketable for those seeking these services. I also found it helpful to start package programs for those who like to buy sessions in bundles where they can receive a discount as opposed to paying for one session at a time. I began to broaden my scope with consultation by also doing them for businesses and individuals. My consultation services included implementation of multicultural systems to attract clients of color as well as supporting therapists of color. I also included training for staff in different companies and agencies as it related to communication and cohesion for staff.

Additionally, within the last year, I included consultation services for individuals interested in incorporating spirituality into their practices and transitioning from a solo to a group practice. I also added supervision mentorship to Dr. Coop Love for those interested in becoming AAMFT (American Association of Marriage and Family Therapists) approved supervisors. As I got more familiar with consultation and supervision, I added dissertation coaching as I felt this was a missing gap for those who needed assistance and support during their dissertation process. For me, this was something I wanted during my doctoral studies and I wanted to provide that to those who needed that type of support. I created package programs for dissertation coaching which includes an intensive 12-month program, 6-month program (to be paid monthly), or a bundle of four coaching sessions.

Separating myself and the consultation services I provided were important in distinguishing between the things suited best for therapy client's vs clients who needed consultation services. Adding Dr. Coop-Love in addition to the ANC business was helpful in separating my work outside of therapy from the therapy practice. I needed a website specific to me and the services that I provided as a consultant, speaker, supervisor, trainer, and coach.

Transition from Solo to Group Practice

I had been a solo private practice for over five years in my business. Over the years, I had potential interns and associates reach out for opportunities to work in my practice, but at the time I did not have the capacity to begin a group practice fully. At the end of 2020, I made the decision to officially become a group practice. COVID had impacted my business to a degree initially because most of my clients still wanted to be seen in person. At the time, this was not an option for me as I was pregnant and due within a couple of months. I knew that I would need more hands to assist in serving clients as there had been a tremendous influx of referrals. As the year went on, I was booked out for almost three months. I knew that I would not have the capacity to see all the clients that were coming in as well as having a newborn baby, it would be too much strain.

As a result, I added four associates who had completed their Master's degrees. I had supervisory relationships with them for a couple of years and we built a great professional relationship together. Since then, I've hired an administrative assistant working part-time to assist in phone calls, systems, protocols, and emails along with one of my associates who is also responsible for handling things on the front-end of the business. It was important for me to add an assistant who had customer service experience as well as currently going to school in the field. I've also recruited undergraduate interns to assist the admin team as well as creating social media posts. This gives them experience with speaking to potential clients as well as marketing through social media and gaining visibility. I've also added a Masters level intern and provided an internship for her in order to gain her practicum hours as an upcoming marriage and family therapist. Having an intern aids in creating affordable therapy for those who could not afford my rates. I transitioned from accepting sliding scale on my caseload and had a team of pre-licensed therapists who could assist in providing affordable therapy services. This also helped us to create a co-payment program where clients are allowed to pay their copay at a minimum of $30 with student interns for up to eight sessions.

I found that adding interns and pre-licensed professionals fit better with my businesses as they are more eager to learn and are proactive when it comes to getting things done, gaining their clients, and fitting well as a team player. As mentioned earlier, having interns and associates providing affordable therapy services benefit clients who cannot pay the market rate. I pride myself in having a team that is cohesive, and can foster an environment of growth and learning from one another. My goal as a supervisor and employer is to assist my associates in flourishing and succeeding beyond ANC. Having a team is helpful when everyone does their part. Since adding the ANC team, we can provide specific services for populations based on associates' specialties as well as conducting groups and other events to ANC services.

Incorporating Spirituality into Mental Health Practice

When incorporating spirituality in mental health practice, our society typically views spirituality and mental health as separate, especially as it relates to sex and sexuality. The infusion of spirituality into the mental health field is contrary to the historical positions of mental health professionals (Ullery, 2004). In 2021, I made the decision to rebrand my practice. I had a pressing thought that my practice could expand beyond therapy. I also had the thought that I was not operating in my full capacity to serve clients beyond the mental and emotional. I was moved to focus on a more holistic perspective that incorporated mind, body, and spirit. I adopted a transpersonal psychotherapy perspective which believes the spirit that needs healing in addition to the mind and the body. I also introduced tantra and heart-work for those interested in that type of healing work in addition to therapy services. I started a separate business for my spiritual practice because I wanted to ensure that the services were from a different entity than ANC. I could operate as a business solely for spiritual work outside of the therapy platform as well. As it relates to ethics, all clients had to complete consent forms which are separate from ANC when it comes to receiving spiritual work.

I believe that tantric healing and heart work marries well with therapy, and it addresses the spirit in addition to emotional, mental, and physical wellness. For many, tantra is a new phenomenon, making many of its concepts and teachings both complex and difficult to understand. Before my certification as a tantric healer, I conducted research on it and the positive impact it has on people's lives. It has been found that tantra aids clients to release their pain through pleasure. It has been known to aid in alleviating infertility, erectile dysfunction, desire, arousal, and orgasmic issues (Morris, 2020). Tantra connects the physical, mental, and emotional with the spiritual; a practice which could aid in reducing sexual issues within self and in relationships.

I have found that doing this work in conjunction with therapy practices aids in the transformation process for clients who have been battling wounds of their past. This would also be beneficial to those who suffered traumatic experiences. These experiences shape how individuals are in relationship with themselves and others. Wolf and Stevens (2001) outlined expected client benefits with a spiritual inclusion in therapy. Possible among these are increased family cohesion, enhanced physical and mental health, increased community support, and improved ethical considerations. When spirituality is incorporated, it is most effective when there is a blend of mind, body, and spirit.

Considerations

As a business owner, there are steps that are pertinent to starting, growing, and maintaining a business. Some things that are helpful to consider is to research as much as possible the state requirements to start and build your private practice. Every state is different and has requirements that may vary from state to state. There is also the importance of distinguishing whether your potential practice is self-paying only or insurance/self-pay. It makes a difference in your marketing, and scripts that you use to speak with clients. It will also affect the initial growth of your practice. I often share the practice of slow and steady. Take your time, read through everything, and do your research. Business coaches are great assets to a business as they help you to see your vision more clearly and give you ideas that fit within your goals. An accountability partner is also crucial in holding you to your own standards and goals to get things done in your business. Knowing your worth as a professional and businessperson will aid in the growing and thriving of your business. Those things are what separate successful businesses from those who are not as successful.

When it comes to incorporating spiritual energy work in your practice (tantra, reiki, etc.). There is the importance of maintaining the balance between therapy practice and spiritual practice. It is imperative to keep the boundaries clear and concise as it relates to healing work from both the spiritual and mental health perspectives. It is also important for the client to have spiritual and religious autonomy and can discuss whatever they deem as necessary during therapy (Wolf & Stevens, 2001). It is crucial to provide a safe and open space for clients to share whatever their issues are from a spiritual and mental, and sexual perspective, and to honor their decisions of whether they want to add spiritual interventions to their treatment. Business ownership is not the easiest thing, however it's the most rewarding thing. Other business owners that I've met over the years all shared the same statement. They all stated that becoming a full-time business owner was the best decision they had ever made in their life. As a full-time business owner, I can attest that this is the truth. Developing a plan, financial system, and support of colleagues are great recipes for starting, maintaining, and growing a successful business.

References

Morris, Y. N. (2020). *The holy grail of orgasm*. Atlanta, GA: Grand Trine Productions.

Truffo, C. (2012). *Be a wealthy therapist: Finally, you can make a living while making a difference*. MP Press: St. Peters, MO.

Ullery, E. K. (2004). Consideration of a spiritual role in sex and sex therapy. *The Family Journal: Counseling and Therapy for Couples and Families*, 12(1), 78–81. DOI:10.1177/1066480703258710

Wolf, C., & Stevens, P. (2001). Integrating religion and spirituality in marriage and family counseling. *Counseling and Values*, 46(1), 66–76.

Index

For Product Safety Concerns and Information please contact our EU
representative GPSR@taylorandfrancis.com
Taylor & Francis Verlag GmbH, Kaufingerstraße 24, 80331 München, Germany

www.ingramcontent.com/pod-product-compliance
Lightning Source LLC
Chambersburg PA
CBHW060255220326
41598CB00027B/4111

* 9 7 8 1 0 3 2 3 2 3 6 5 7 *